SYSTEMS THINKING

for Health Systems Strengthening

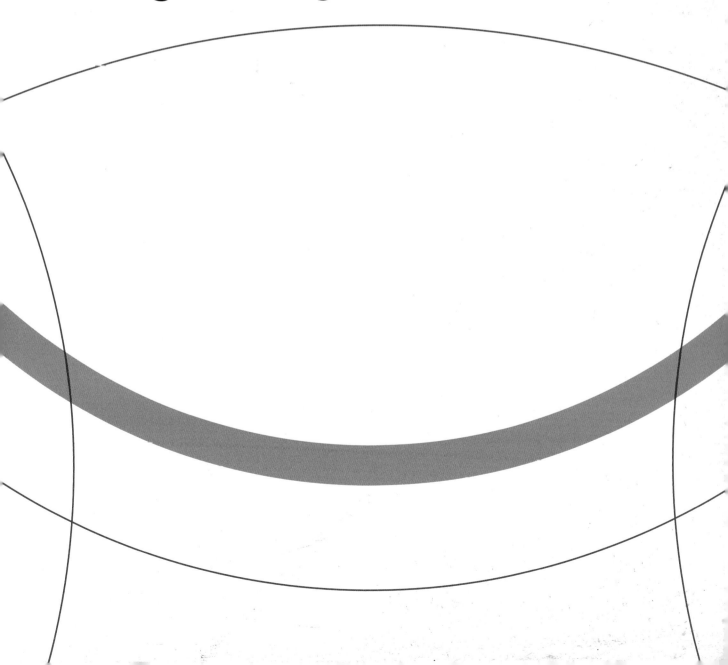

WHO Library Cataloguing-in-Publication Data

Systems thinking for health systems strengthening / edited by Don de Savigny and Taghreed Adam.

1.Delivery of health care – organization and administration. 2.Delivery of health care – trends. 3.Systems theory. 4.Health services research. 5.Cooperative behavior. 6.Health policy. I.de Savigny, Donald. II.Adam, Taghreed. III.Alliance for Health Policy and Systems Research. IV.World Health Organization.

ISBN 978 92 4 156389 5   (NLM classification: W 84)

Printed in France
Designed by Capria
Design Consultant: James B. Williams
Suggested citation: Don de Savigny and Taghreed Adam (Eds). Systems thinking for health systems strengthening. Alliance for Health Policy and Systems Research, WHO, 2009.

Contents

Contents

Chapter 1

Chapter 2

Chapter 3

Chapter 4

Systems thinking for health systems: Challenges and opportunities in real-world settings

Chapter 5

Systems thinking for health systems strengthening: Moving forward

List of Figures

List of Tables

List of Boxes

List of Boxes (CONTINUED)

Acknowledgments

Acknowledgments

This Flagship Report is the joint product of a number of people, and the Alliance wishes to thank them for their input.

Editors: Don de Savigny and Taghreed Adam

Principal authors:

Chapter 1. *Systems thinking for health systems strengthening: An introduction*
Don de Savigny and Taghreed Adam

Chapter 2. *Systems thinking: What it is and what it means for health systems*
Don de Savigny, Taghreed Adam, Sandy Campbell and Allan Best

Chapter 3. *Systems thinking: Applying a systems perspective to design and evaluate health systems interventions*
Don de Savigny, Josephine Borghi, Ricarda Windisch, Alan Shiell and Taghreed Adam

Chapter 4. *Systems thinking for health systems: Challenges and opportunities in real-world settings*
Taghreed Adam, Sangeeta Mookherji, Sandy Campbell, Graham Reid, Lucy Gilson and Don de Savigny

Chapter 5. *Systems thinking for health systems strengthening: Moving forward*
Don de Savigny

Web Annex. *Evaluation of interventions with system-wide effects in developing countries: Exploratory review*
(http://www.who.int/alliance-hpsr/resources/en/)
Dominique Guinot, Barbara Koloshuk, Kaspar Wyss and Taghreed Adam

Valuable technical inputs and review comments were provided by various people through participation at a brainstorming workshop (September 2008), an experts consultation meeting (April 2009) and reviewing chapter drafts (in alphabetical order):

Irene Agyepong	Sennen Hounton	Mark Petticrew
Anwer Aqil	Aklilu Kidanu	Kent Ranson
Sara Bennett	Soonman Kwon	Graham Reid
Allan Best	Mary Ann Lansang	John-Arne Röttingen
David Bishai	John Lavis	Sarah Russel
Valerie Crowell	Daniel Low-Beer	Alan Shiell
Marjolein Dieleman	Prasanta Mahapatra	Terry Smutylo
Shams El-Arifeen	Lindiwe Makubalo	Göran Tomson
David Evans	Anne Mills	Phyllida Travis
Lucy Gilson	David Peters	Cesar Victora

Sandy Campbell was copy editor and Lydia Al Khudri managed the production of the report.

Preface

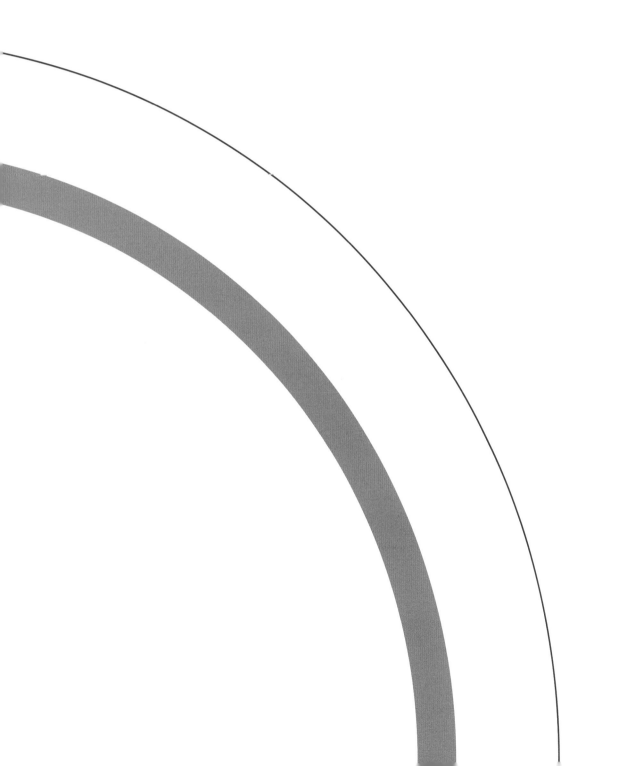

Preface

Strong health systems are fundamental if we are to improve health outcomes and accelerate progress towards the Millennium Development Goals of reducing maternal and child mortality, and combating HIV, malaria and other diseases. At a time when economic downturn, a new influenza pandemic, and climate change add to the challenges of meeting those goals, the need for robust health systems is more acute than ever.

Often, however, health system strengthening seems a distant, even abstract aim. This should not and need not be the case.

I therefore welcome this Flagship Report from the Alliance for Health Policy and Systems Research, which offers a fresh and practical approach to strengthening health systems through "systems thinking". This powerful tool first decodes the complexity of a health system, and then applies that understanding to design better interventions to strengthen systems, increase coverage, and improve health.

In its "Ten Steps to Systems Thinking," this Report shows how we can better capture the wisdom of diverse stakeholders in designing solutions to system problems. It suggests ways to more realistically forecast how health systems might respond to strengthening interventions, while also exploring potential synergies and dangers among those interventions. Lastly, it shows how better evaluations of health system strengthening initiatives can yield valuable lessons about what works, how it works and for whom.

Health systems strengthening is rising on political agendas worldwide. Precise and nuanced knowledge and understanding of what constitutes an effective health system is growing all the time – a phenomenon that is well reflected in this Report. This Flagship Report will deepen understanding and stimulate fresh thinking among stewards of health systems, health systems researchers, and development partners. I look forward to seeing its results.

Dr Margaret Chan
Director-General, World Health Organization, Geneva
November 2009

Executive Summary

Executive Summary

The Problem

Despite strong global consensus on the need to strengthen health systems, there is no established framework for doing so in developing countries, and no formula to apply or package of interventions to implement. Many health systems simply lack the capacity to measure or understand their own weaknesses and constraints, which effectively leaves policy-makers without scientifically sound ideas of what they can and should actually strengthen. Within such unmapped and misunderstood systems, interventions – even the very simplest – often fail to achieve their goals. This is not necessarily due to any inherent flaw in the intervention itself but rather to the often unpredictable behaviour of the system around it. *Every intervention, from the simplest to the most complex, has an effect on the overall system, and the overall system has an effect on every intervention.*

As investments in health are expanded in low- and middle-income countries, and as funders increasingly support broader initiatives for health system strengthing, we need to know not only what works but what works for whom and under what circumstances. If we accept that no intervention is simple, and that every act of intervening has effects – intended and unintended – across the system, then it is imperative that we begin to understand the full range of those effects in order to mitigate any negative behaviour and to amplify any possible synergies. We must know the system in order to strengthen it – and from that base we can design better interventions and evaluations, for both health systems strengthening interventions and for interventions targeting specific diseases or conditions but with the potential of having system-wide effects.

How we design those interventions and evaluate their effects is the challenge at the heart of this Report.

Systems Thinking

To understand and appreciate the relationships within systems, several recent projects have adopted systems thinking to tackle complex health problems and risk factors – in tobacco control, obesity and tuberculosis. On a broader level, however, systems thinking has huge and untapped potential, first in deciphering the complexity of an entire health system, and then in applying this understanding to design and evaluate interventions that improve health and health equity. Systems thinking can provide a way forward for operating more successfully and effectively in complex, real-world settings. It can open powerful pathways to identifying and resolving health system challenges, and as such is a crucial ingredient for any health system strengthening effort.

Systems thinking works to reveal the underlying characteristics and relationships of systems. Work in fields as diverse as engineering, economics and ecology shows systems to be constantly changing, with components that are tightly connected and highly sensitive to change elsewhere in the system. They are non-linear, unpredictable and resistant to change, with seemingly obvious solutions sometimes worsening a problem. Systems are dynamic architectures of interactions and synergies. WHO's framework of health system building blocks effectively describes six sub-systems of an overall health system architecture. Anticipating how an intervention might flow through, react with, and impinge on these sub-systems is crucial and forms the opportunity to apply systems thinking in a constructive way.

Applying Systems Thinking

Systems thinking provides a deliberate and comprehensive suite of tools and approaches to map, measure and understand these dynamics. In this Report, we propose "Ten Steps to Systems Thinking" for real-world guidance in applying such an approach in the health system. We use a major contemporary health financing intervention as a case illustration to demonstrate how a broad partnership of stakeholders can deliver a richer understanding of the implications of the intervention, including how the system will react, respond and change, along with what synergies can be harnessed, and what negative emergent behaviour should be mitigated. We can then apply this understanding to a safer and more robust intervention design and an evaluation that goes beyond the usual "input-blackbox-output" paradigm to one that accounts for system behaviour. The systems thinking approach connects intervention design and evaluation more explicitly, both to each other and to the health system framework.

TEN STEPS TO SYSTEMS THINKING IN THE HEALTH SYSTEM

I. Intervention Design	II. Evaluation Design
1. Convene stakeholders	5. Determine indicators
2. Collectively brainstorm	6. Choose methods
3. Conceptualize effects	7. Select design
4. Adapt and redesign	8. Develop plan
	9. Set budget
	10. Source funding.

Challenges, Opportunities and Moving Forward

Many practitioners may dismiss systems thinking as too complicated or unsuited for any practical purpose or application. While the pressures and dynamics of actual situations may block or blur the systems perspective, we argue that the timing for applying such an approach has never been better. Many developing countries are looking to scale-up "what works" through major systems strengthening investments. With leadership, conviction and commitment, systems thinking can accelerate the strengthening of systems better able to produce health with equity and deliver interventions to those in need.

Systems thinking is not a panacea. Its application does not mean that resolving problems and weaknesses will come easily or naturally or without overcoming the inertia of the established way of doing things. But it will identify, with more precision, where some of the true blockages and challenges lie. It will help to:

1) explore these problems from a systems perspective;

2) show potentials of solutions that work across sub-systems;

3) promote dynamic networks of diverse stakeholders;

4) inspire learning; and

5) foster more system-wide planning, evaluation and research.

And it will increase the likelihood that health system strengthening investments and interventions will be effective. The more often and more comprehensively the actors and components of the system can talk to each other from within a common framework — communicating, sharing, problem-solving — the better chance any initiative to strengthen health systems has. Real progress will undoubtedly require time, significant change, and momentum to build capacity across the system. However, the change is necessary — and needed now.

The Report therefore speaks to health system stewards, researchers, and funders. It maps out a set of strategies and activities to harness systems thinking approaches, to link them to these emerging opportunities, and to promote systems thinking as the norm in the design and evaluation of interventions in health systems.

But, the final message is to the funders of health system strengthening and health systems research who will need to recognize the potential in these opportunities, be prepared to take risks in investing in such innovations, and play an active role in both driving and following this agenda towards more systemic and evidence-informed health development.

Acronyms

Acronyms

AHPSR	Alliance for Health Policy and Systems Research
ANC	Ante-natal Care
ART	Anti-retroviral Therapy
CCT	Conditional Cash Transfer
COHRED	Council on Health Research for Development
DECIPHer	Centre for the Development and Evaluation of Complex Interventions for Public Health Improvement
EPI	Expanded Programme for Immunization
FGDs	Focus Group Discussions
HIC	High-Income Country
HIS	Health Information System
HIV/AIDS	Human Immunodeficiency Virus / Acquired Immunodeficiency Syndrome
HMIS	Health Management Information System
HMN	Health Metrics Network
HSR	Health Systems Research
IMCI	Integrated Management of Childhood Illnesses
IIN	Insecticide-treated Mosquito Net
LMIC	Low- and Middle-income Country
MDGs	Millennium Development Goals
P4P	Pay-for-Performance (called both pay- and paying-for-performance in Chapter 3)
PAHO	Pan American Health Organization
PBF	Performance-based Funding
PHC	Primary Health Care
RCTs	Randomized Controlled Trials
SES	Socio-economic Status
ST	Systems Thinking
SWAps	Sector-wide Approaches
TB DOTS	Directly Observed Treatment for Tuberculosis – short course
TNVS	Tanzania National Voucher Scheme
UNDP	United Nations Development Programme
UNICEF	United Nations Children's Fund
WB	World Bank
WHO	World Health Organization

1

Systems thinking for health systems strengthening: An introduction

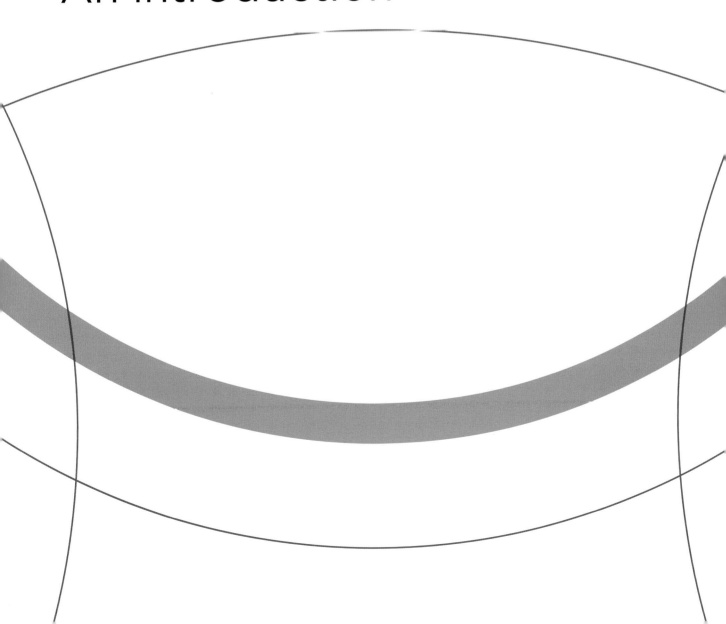

Flagship Report Series

The Alliance for Health Policy and Systems Research ("the Alliance") is an international collaboration based within WHO Geneva. Its primary goal is to promote the generation and use of health policy and systems research as a means to improve health and health systems in developing countries. The Alliance's *Flagship Report Series* is a key instrument in promoting innovative ideas that address current gaps or challenges and stimulating debate on a priority topic identified by stakeholders in the field.

The first Flagship Report was 2004's "Strengthening health systems: the role and promise of policy and systems research," with the principal goal of increasing knowledge on health systems and applying that knowledge to strengthen health systems. The second Report, produced in 2007, was "Sound Choices: enhancing capacity for evidence-informed health policy," which analyzed capacity constraints in linking research and policy processes. This third Report knits together the earlier work by accelerating a more realistic understanding of what works in strengthening health systems, for whom, and under what circumstances. Its primary goal is to catalyze new conceptual thinking on health systems, system-level interventions, and health system strengthening.

"For the first time, public health has commitment, resources, and powerful interventions. What is missing is this. The power of these interventions is not matched by the power of health systems to deliver them to those in greatest need, on an adequate scale, in time. This lack of capacity arises ... in part, from the fact that research on health systems has been so badly neglected and underfunded."
Dr Margaret Chan, Director-General, WHO. 29 October 2007

Introduction to the Report

The challenges of meeting the Millennium Development Goals (MDGs) for health remain formidable. While the current decade has seen significant advances in the health sector of low- and middle-income countries, this progress has been slower than expected (1). Despite a strong range of health interventions that can prevent much of the burden of disease in the poorest countries – with ever-improving interventions in the pipeline – effective coverage of these interventions is expanding too slowly (2;3) and health inequities are widening (4). Cost-effective interventions – when available – are both inadequately provided and underused (1).

In many cases, the fundamental problem lies with the broader health system and its ability to deliver interventions to those who need them. Weaknesses and obstacles exist across the system, including overall stewardship and management issues; critical supply-side issues such as human resources, infrastructure, information, and service provision; and demand-side issues such as people's participation, knowledge and behaviour (5;6). Even more, specific losses in health intervention efficacy due to health systems delivery issues are often grossly underestimated (7).

BOX 1.1 GOALS OF THIS REPORT

Over 2008, wide global consultation revealed considerable interest and frustration among researchers, funders and policy-makers around our limited understanding of what works in health systems strengthening. In this current *Flagship Report* we introduce and discuss the merits of employing a systems thinking approach in order to catalyze conceptual thinking regarding health systems, system-level interventions, and evaluations of health system strengthening. The Report sets out to answer the following broad questions:

■ What is systems thinking and how can researchers and policy-makers apply it?

■ How can we use this perspective to better understand and exploit the synergies among interventions to strengthen health systems?

■ How can systems thinking contribute to better evaluations of these system-level interventions?

This Report argues that a stronger systems perspective among designers, implementers, stewards and funders is a critical component in strengthening overall health-sector development in low- and middle-income countries.

Systemic factors and their effects are poorly studied and evaluated. Few health systems have the capacity to measure or understand their strengths and weaknesses, especially in regard to equity, effectiveness and their respective determinants. Without this broader understanding of a system's capacity, the research and development community struggles to design specific interventions that optimize the health system's ability to deliver essential health interventions. And – crucially – all too often there is another poorly appreciated phenomenon: *every health intervention, from the simplest to the most complex, has an effect on the overall system*. Presumably simple interventions targeting one health system entry point have multiple and sometimes counter-intuitive effects elsewhere in the system. Even when we anticipate the system-wide effects of multi-faceted and complex interventions, our approaches to charting, evaluating and understanding them are often weak and sometimes entirely absent. It is increasingly clear that no intervention – with a particular emphasis on system-level or system-wide interventions – ought to be considered "simple".

It is imperative that we understand the complex effects, synergies[1] and emergent behaviour of system interventions in order to capitalize on the current momentum of building stronger health systems (8). As investments in health are expanded and as funders increasingly support broader initiatives for health system strengthening, we need to know not only what works but for whom, and under what circumstances (9-17).

How we design interventions and evaluate effects, for both health systems strengthening interventions and for interventions targeting specific health diseases or conditions are the challenges at the heart of this Report. We argue throughout that a systems thinking approach can greatly benefit overall health-sector development.

How we design interventions and evaluate effects, for both health systems strengthening interventions and for interventions targeting specific diseases or conditions, are the challenges at the heart of this Report.

It has huge potential, first in decoding the complexity of a health system, and then in using this understanding to design and evaluate interventions that maximize health and health equity. System thinking can provide a way forward for operating more successfully and effectively in complex, real-world settings. It can open powerful pathways to identifying and resolving health system challenges, and as such is a crucial ingredient for any health system strengthening effort.

Key terms and terminology

Arriving first at a clear set of concepts and terminology is essential, and to that end we discuss below the key terms used throughout this Report: the health system, health system building blocks, "people," systems thinking, system-level interventions, and evaluation.

The Health System. Following the definition of the World Health Organization, a health system *"consists of all organizations, people and actions whose primary intent is to promote, restore or maintain health"* (5). Its goals are *"improving health and health equity in ways that are responsive, financially fair, and make the best, or most efficient, use of available resources"* (5).

In referring to the individual components of health systems, this Report uses the current WHO "Framework for Action" on health systems, which describes six clearly defined **Health System Building Blocks** that together constitute a complete system (5). Throughout this Report, these building blocks serve as a convenient device for exploring the health

---

[1] A "synergy" is a situation where different entities combine advantageously – where the whole becomes greater than the sum of the individual parts.

system and understanding the effects of interventions upon it. These building blocks are:

- *Service delivery:* including effective, safe, and quality personal and non-personal health interventions that are provided to those in need, when and where needed (including infrastructure), with a minimal waste of resources;

- *Health workforce:* responsive, fair and efficient given available resources and circumstances, and available in sufficient numbers;

- *Health information:* ensuring the production, analysis, dissemination and use of reliable and timely information on health determinants, health systems performance and health status;

- *Medical technologies:* including medical products, vaccines and other technologies of assured quality, safety, efficacy and cost-effectiveness, and their scientifically sound and cost-effective use;

- *Health financing:* raising adequate funds for health in ways that ensure people can use needed services, and are protected from financial catastrophe or impoverishment associated with having to pay for them;

- *Leadership and governance:* ensuring strategic policy frameworks combined with effective oversight, coalition building, accountability, regulations, incentives and attention to system design.

The building blocks alone do not constitute a system, any more than a pile of bricks constitutes a functioning building (Figure 1.1). It is the multiple relationships and interactions among the blocks – how one affects and influences the others, and is in turn affected by them – that convert these blocks into a system (Figure 1.2). As such, a health system may be understood through the arrangement and interaction of its parts, and how they enable the system to achieve the purpose for which it was designed (5).

The building blocks alone do not constitute a system, any more than a pile of bricks constitutes a functioning building. It is the multiple relationships and interactions among the blocks – how one affects and influences the others, and is in turn affected by them – that convert these blocks into a system.

Figure 1.1   The building blocks of the health system: aims and attributes (5)

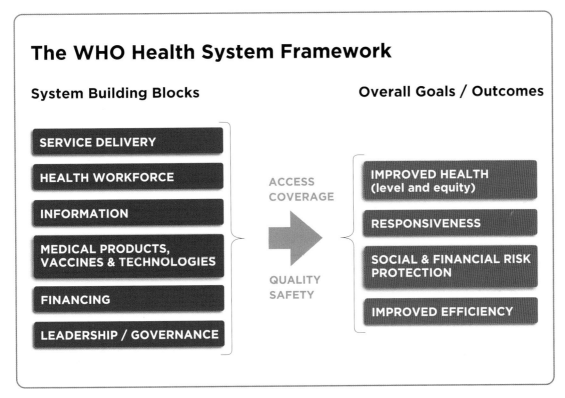

The health system building blocks are sub-systems of the health system that function – and therefore must be understood – together in a dynamic architecture of interactions and synergies.

Health systems are often seen as monolithic, as a macro system with little attention paid to the interaction among its component parts, when in fact they are a dynamo of interactions, synergies and shifting sub-systems. If we see the building blocks as sub-systems of the health system, we see that within every sub-system is an array of other systems. All systems are contained or "nested" within larger systems (18;19). Within the heath system is the sub-system for service delivery; within that system may be a hospital system, and within that a laboratory system; and among all of these sub-systems are reactions, synergies and interactions to varying degrees with all of the health system's other building blocks.

People. It is critical that the role of people is highlighted, not just at the centre of the system as mediators and beneficiaries but as actors in driving the system itself. This includes their participation as individuals, civil society organizations, and stakeholder networks, and also as key actors influencing each of the building blocks, as health workers, managers and policy-makers. Placing people and their institutions in the centre of this framework emphasizes WHO's renewed commitment to the principles and values of primary health care – fairness, social justice, participation and inter-sectoral collaboration (20;21).

Figure 1.2   The dynamic architecture and interconnectedness of the health system building blocks

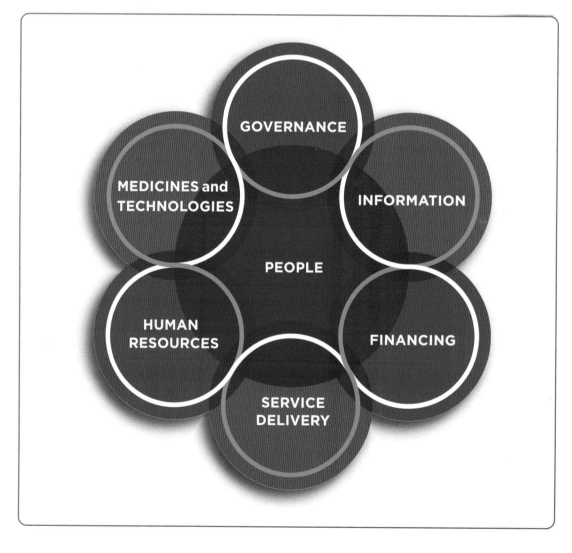

Systems thinking is an approach to problem solving that views "problems" as part of a wider, dynamic system. Systems thinking involves much more than a reaction to present outcomes or events. It demands a deeper understanding of the linkages, relationships, interactions and behaviours among the elements that characterize the entire system. Commonly used in other sectors where interventions and systems are complex, systems thinking in the health sector shifts the focus to:

- the nature of relationships among the building blocks

- the spaces between the blocks (and understanding what happens there)

- the synergies emerging from interactions among the blocks.

The application of systems thinking in the health sector is accelerating a more realistic understanding of what works, for whom, and under what circumstances (22-24).

Interventions with system-wide effects and system-level interventions. All health

interventions have system-level effects to a greater or lesser degree on one or more of the system's building blocks. Many may be relatively simple interventions or incremental changes to existing interventions – e.g. adding vitamin A supplementation to routine vaccination – and not all interventions will benefit from or need a systems thinking approach. However, more complex interventions – e.g. the scaling-up of antiretroviral therapy – can be expected to have profound effects across the system, especially in weaker health systems (Figure 1.3) (25;26). They thus require a systems thinking approach to illuminate the full range of effects and potential synergies. This Report refers to these as "interventions with system-wide effects".

"System-level interventions" target one or multiple system building blocks directly or generically (e.g. human resources for health), rather than a health problem specifically. Given their effects on other building blocks, "system-level interventions" strongly benefit from a systems thinking approach. As explored in detail in Chapter 3 of this Report, a financing instrument such as paying-for-performance is a "system-level intervention" as it will affect almost all other building blocks of the health system. It will for example present **governance** challenges around the accountability and transparency concerning bonus payments dispensed to staff in health facilities; affect the **information** system in tracking and reconciling the conditions triggering cash payments; strongly influence **service delivery** by changing staff behaviour, increasing utilization, or possibly crowding-out other services; might conflict with other **financing** modalities, potentially running counter to sector-wide and budget support

More complex interventions can be expected to have profound effects across the system, especially in weaker health systems

approaches; and it may also shape **human resources** by improving (or eroding) provider motivation.

A systems thinking approach will help to anticipate and mitigate such effects when developing interventions, as well as harnessing unexpected synergies by modifying the interventions. This then provides the basis for understanding how to measure them in better designed and more comprehensive evaluations.

Evaluation. The conventional evaluation of inputs, outcomes and impacts can only take us so far, often failing to illuminate the key determinants and contexts that explain overall success or create particular difficulties. Funders and programmes seeking to understand and evaluate their investments and inputs tend to focus more on downstream disease and mortality impacts. As a result, they often neglect the wider health system synergies and emergent behaviour that might, in the end, be more

instructive in terms of the systems strengthening necessary to achieve the health goals. Such approaches to evaluation often inhibit the broader systems perspective and a fuller understanding of how interventions do or do not work, for whom, and under what conditions.

The systems thinking approach goes beyond this "input-blackbox-output" paradigm to one that considers inputs, outputs, initial, intermediate and eventual outcomes, *and* feedback, processes, flows, control and contexts (22). Given that all evaluations are necessary simplifications of real-world complexity, systems thinking helps to determine how much – and where – to simplify. A systems thinking approach can connect intervention design and evaluation more explicitly, both to each other and to the health system framework – though it should be added that not all interventions require evaluation or evaluation with a systems thinking lens (see Figure 1.3).

Figure 1.3 A spectrum of interventions and their potential for system-wide effects

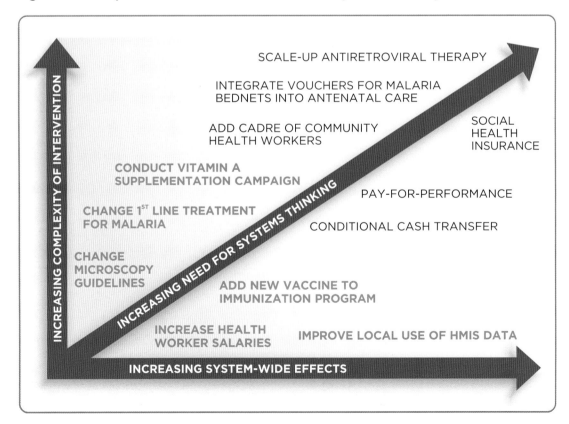

BOX 1.3 INDICATORS AND TOOLS FOR MONITORING CHANGES IN HEALTH SYSTEMS

Interventions designed to strengthen the system – and their evaluations – often undervalue the need to understand, strengthen and evaluate the relationships among the system's building blocks. Work to develop sensitive and easily measurable indicators for monitoring changes within each health system building block is ongoing. Such tools are necessary if systems are to become capable of achieving the effective and universal coverage – at sufficient quality and safety – necessary for improved health and health equity, responsiveness, risk protection and efficiency.

For more on these indicators and tools, see WHO 2009 Draft Toolkit for Strengthening Health Systems. Available at: http://www.who.int/healthinfo/statistics/toolkit_hss/en/index.html

Overview of the Report

We pursue several goals in this Report. Its primary goal is to catalyze new conceptual thinking on health systems, system-level interventions, and health system strengthening. For this we introduce systems thinking and show how it might improve intervention design and evaluation by more careful consideration of system-wide effects. We explore the scientific foundations for this, providing both a conceptual and an operational approach to designing and evaluating interventions with a systems perspective. This includes illustrating important on-going challenges and proposing practical steps, while also reinforcing advocacy for funding and conducting evaluations of health systems strengthening interventions.

In Chapter 2, we introduce and explore systems thinking and what it means for the health system as an overall primer to the issues and relevant literature. The chapter is targeted to all audiences (including system stewards, intervention designers, researchers, evaluators, and funding partners).

While retaining a rigorous scientific base, systems thinking requires us to go beyond cause-and-effect approaches. Primarily aimed at intervention designers and evaluators, Chapter 3 introduces the scientific rationale for evaluations that take a systems perspective and illustrates – in ten steps – how interventions with a system-wide impact could be better designed and evaluated. This includes guidance for developing conceptual frameworks and understanding system-wide implications, and an overview of relevant intervention design and evaluation questions, choice of indicators, and how to match evaluation designs to intervention designs. This chapter is further informed by the nature and gaps in recent evaluations of system-level interventions (reviewed as a background to this Report, with a summary of findings available in the Web Annex at http://www.who.int/alliance-hpsr/resources/en/).

Of course, applying a systems thinking perspective is far from straightforward, marked by as many challenges as opportunities. It can, for instance, enhance a more inclusive participatory approach that fosters direct links to policy-making, and better ownership of processes and outcomes. It can build national capacity in solving health system problems and facilitate use of research evidence to inform policy-making.

But it can also run counter to dominant paradigms and relationships. The complex dynamics among the public, researchers, programme implementers, funders and political agents pose many challenges to the systems perspective. We explore some of these implications and provide examples of how they have been experienced or managed in Chapter 4. This Chapter mainly targets system stewards, evaluators, and funding partners.

Finally, Chapter 5 reflects on the way forward for systems thinking for health systems strengthening and provides a set of ideas for various stakeholders.

As with all system-oriented problems, the issues and approaches discussed here are inherently intricate and not always intuitive. Our Report attempts to make the case for a broader systems thinking approach in an easily accessible form for a broad interdisciplinary audience, including health system stewards, programme implementers, researchers, evaluators and funding partners. It is hoped that this Report will stimulate and legitimize more carefully considered funding for better interventions for health systems strengthening and their evaluation as well as fresh thinking, broader approaches, and research that respects and informs the systems approach.

2

Systems thinking:
What it is and what it means
for health systems

Key messages

- Using a systems perspective to understand how health system building blocks, contexts, and actors act, react and interact with each other is an essential approach in designing and evaluating interventions.

- Mainstreaming a stronger systems perspective in the health sector will assist this understanding and accelerate health system strengthening.

- Systems thinking offers a comprehensive way of anticipating synergies and mitigating negative emergent behaviours, with direct relevance for creating policies that are more system-ready.

"The responses of many health systems so far have been generally considered inadequate and naïve. Inadequate, insofar as they not only fail to anticipate, but also to respond appropriately – too often with too little, too late, or too much in the wrong place. Naïve insofar as a system's failure requires a system's solution – not a temporary remedy."
WHO World Health Report, 2008.

Objectives of the Chapter

Systems thinking is an essential approach for strengthening health systems, particularly in designing and evaluating interventions. Chapter 1 described the current WHO framework for action in strengthening health systems, a single people-centered framework combining six clearly defined building blocks or sub-systems (5). However, despite the rising prominence (and sometimes rhetoric) of health systems strengthening among governments and funders, there is little guidance on how to do so. Many subsequent programmes and evaluations still ignore the fundamental characteristics of systems, often considering the individual building blocks in isolation rather than as part of a dynamic whole. Conceptualizing the synergies, intended or not, of intervening in the health system depends upon a fuller understanding of the "system," and how its component parts act, react and interact with each other in an often counter-intuitive process of connectivity and change. As a primer to the issues and relevant literature, this chapter discusses system characteristics and the paradigm shift of systems thinking for strengthening health systems.

Systems thinking

Systems thinking has its origins in the early 20th century in fields as diverse as engineering, economics and ecology. With the increasing emergence of complexity, these and other non-health disciplines developed systems thinking to understand and appreciate the relationships within any given system, and in designing and evaluating system-level interventions (18;27-33). In recent years, the health sector has started to adopt systems thinking to tackle complex sectoral problems such as tobacco control (22), obesity (34-36), and tuberculosis (37). However, few have tried to implement these concepts beyond single issues to the health system itself, or described how to move from theory to practice (18;27) – perhaps due to the seemingly overwhelming complexity of any given health system (29;38-40).

More recently, the suggestion of applying systems thinking to the health system has emerged (41), assisted in some ways by the WHO's 2007 articulation of the health system building blocks (see Chapter 1 for an introduction to this). Although that framework may be challenged as tilted towards supply-side inputs, it does provide a valuable device for conceptualizing the health system and appreciating the utility of systems thinking.

BOX 2.1   COMMON SYSTEMS CHARACTERISTICS

Most systems, including health systems, are:

- Self-organizing
- Constantly changing
- Tightly linked
- Governed by feedback

- Non-linear
- History dependent
- Counter-intuitive
- Resistant to change

Compiled and adapted from Sterman, 2006 and Meadows et al, 1982 (32;42)

Bringing the system into focus with a systems thinking lens

Understanding the fundamental characteristics of systems is crucial to seeing how systems work.[2] The characteristics described in Box 2.1 influence – especially when taken together – how systems, including health systems, respond to external factors or to an intervention.

Self-organizing – *system dynamics arise spontaneously from internal structure.* No individual agent or element determines the nature of the system – the organization of a system arises through the dynamic interaction among the system's agents, and through the system's interaction with other

systems (Box 2.2). The building block framework shows how the nature, dynamics and behaviour of health systems is shaped by the multiple and complex interactions among the blocks – and not by the behaviour of any one block alone. For example, weak stewardship structures (the leadership and governance building block) often disregard or ignore valuable communication and feedback (the health information building block), leading to policies and practices that do not adequately respond to the latest information or evidence. The internal structure and organization – marked in this case by a weak or malfunctioning link between the governance and information blocks – influences to a great degree the functions and abilities of the system itself.

BOX 2.2 SYSTEM BEHAVIOUR

"A system to a large extent causes its own behaviour. Once we see the relationship between structure and behaviour, we can begin to understand how systems work, what makes them produce poor results, and how to shift them into better behaviour patterns. System structure is the source of system behaviour. System behaviour reveals itself as a series of events over time" (43).

---

[2] Our definition of "system" is described in the literature as a "complex adaptive system" – one that self-organizes, adapts and evolves with time. "Complexity" arises from a system's interconnected parts, and "adaptivity" from its ability to communicate and change based on experience (22;38).

Constantly changing – *systems adjust and readjust at many interactive time scales.* Change is a constant in all sustainable systems. Indeed, systems that do not change ultimately collapse since they are part of wider systems that do. As systems are adaptive rather than static, they have the ability to generate their own behaviour; to react differently to the same inputs in unpredictable ways; and to evolve in varying ways through interconnections with other parts of the system (which in turn are constantly changing). This element of change and adaptation poses particular and often hidden challenges in evaluating or understanding discrete health systems interventions. Given those constant interactions and the impossibility of freezing individual dynamics, interventions and their effects can hardly be fully understood or effectively measured in isolation from other system building blocks. For example, in a hospital (a sub-system of the service delivery block), reducing the length of stay in one ward may result in increased re-admission rates in another part, compromising quality and costs (41).

Tightly-linked – *the high degree of connectivity means that change in one sub-system affects the others.* Related to the characteristic of change and adaptation is the notion that any intervention targeting one building block will have certain effects (positive and negative) on other building blocks. For instance, introducing a universal health insurance scheme to protect households from high or unexpected health expenditures may lead to the increased utilization of services that patients may otherwise not choose to use if they had to pay for them. Anticipating these positive and negative effects within a context of inter-connection is key to designing and evaluating an intervention over time. Without a systematic framework to consider possible major synergies (or negative emergent behaviour), the less obvious effects of an intervention may be missed, either at the design or evaluation phase (44).

Governed by feedback – *a positive or negative response that may alter the intervention or expected effects.* Systems are controlled by "feedback loops" that provide information flows on the state of the system, moderating behaviour as elements react and "back-react" on each other. One such example is the change of provider practice patterns (44). This adaptation and change of behaviour among providers requires monitoring, evaluating and the design of new mechanisms (within the information block, for instance) to counteract potential negative effects over time.

Non-linearity – *relationships within a system cannot be arranged along a simple input-output line.* System-level interventions are typically non-linear and unpredictable, with their effects often disproportional or distantly related to the original actions and intentions. For instance, interventions to increase quality of care are likely to succeed initially, but as skills reach a certain level or caseloads increase beyond what health workers will accept, the quality-enhancing effects of the intervention may flatten or actually decrease over time (45).

Anticipating positive and negative effects within a context of interconnection is key to designing and evaluating an intervention over time.

History dependent – *short-term effects of intervening may differ from long-term effects.* Time delays are under-appreciated forces affecting systems. For example, community health insurance schemes intending to generate resources to improve the quality of primary health services may fail to generate sufficient initial resources to drive quality change. This could lead to dissatisfaction and the potential collapse of the intervention before coverage can reach the critical thresholds to actually improve services (46). Interventions designed to change people's behaviour require measuring the intervention effects over a longer period of time to avoid making incorrect conclusions of no or limited effects.

Counter-intuitive – *cause and effect are often distant in time and space, defying solutions that pit causes close to the effects they seek to address.* Some apparently simple and effective interventions may not work in some settings – while functioning perfectly well in others. For example, providing a conditional cash transfer to communities to encourage them to seek care may only work effectively in settings where transport and access to those services is affordable, but not elsewhere. Furthermore, such an intervention may dramatically increase utilization with the risk of overwhelming services that were not strengthened in parallel.

Resistant to change – *seemingly obvious solutions may fail or worsen the situation.* Given the above characteristics of systems, and the complexity of their many interactions, it is sometimes difficult and delicate to develop *a priori* an effective policy without a highly astute understanding of the system. System characteristics can render the system "policy resistant," particularly when all of the actors

within a system have their own, and often competing, goals (43). For example, a conditional cash transfer designed to change or increase health-seeking behaviour may in fact worsen the existing situation through the rise of unintended behaviours (e.g. mothers keeping children malnourished to maintain eligibility).

> **BOX 2.3 THE CONNECTIONS AND CONSEQUENCES OF SYSTEMS THINKING**
>
> Systems thinking places high value on understanding context and looking for connections between the parts, actors and processes of the system (Lucy Gilson, personal communication) (48). They make deliberate attempts to anticipate, rather than react to, the downstream consequences of changes in the system, and to identify upstream points of leverage (David Peters, personal communication) (35;49-51). None of this is unfamiliar to those working in health systems, but what is different in systems thinking the deliberate, continuous and comprehensive way in which the approach is applied (22).

Interventions designed to change people's behaviour require measuring the intervention effects over a longer period of time to avoid making incorrect conclusions of no or limited effects.

Systems thinking offers a more comprehensive way of anticipating synergies and mitigating negative emergent behaviours, with direct relevance for creating more system-ready policies.

Systems thinking – a paradigm shift

Given these complex relationships and characteristics of the health system, applying conventional approaches commonly used to design and evaluate interventions will not take us far enough. These approaches are usually described in linear input-output-outcome-impact chains which drive the log-frames characteristically underpinning the monitoring and evaluation of programmes and investments (47). We need a radical shift in the intervention design and evaluation approaches for health systems (37;48), along with anaccompanying shift in mindset among designers, implementers, stewards and funders.

The type of skills needed for system thinking – and the required shift in the way of thinking – are illustrated in Table 2. 1, comparing the more usual with the systems thinking approach.

Table 2.1 Skills of systems thinking

Usual approach	Systems thinking approach
Static thinking	**Dynamic thinking**
Focusing on particular events	Framing a problem in terms of a pattern of behaviour over time
Systems-as-effect thinking	**System-as-cause thinking**
Viewing behaviour generated by a system as driven by external forces	Placing responsibility for a behaviour on internal actors who manage the policies and "plumbing" of the system
Tree-by-tree thinking	**Forest thinking**
Believing that really knowing something means focusing on the details	Believing that to know something requires understanding the context of relationships
Factors thinking	**Operational thinking**
Listing factors that influence or correlate with some result	Concentrating on causality and under-standing how a behaviour is generated
Straight-line thinking	**Loop thinking**
Viewing causality as running in one direction, ignoring (either deliberately or not) the interdependence and interaction between and among the causes	Viewing causality as an on-going process, not a one-time event, with effect feeding back to influence the causes and the causes affecting each other

Modified from Richmond, 2000 (28).

System stakeholder networks

Another vital aspect of systems thinking revolves around how system stakeholder networks are included, composed and managed, and how context shapes this stakeholder behaviour. Stakeholders are not only at the centre of the system as mediators and beneficiaries but are also actors driving the system itself. This includes their participation as individuals, civil society organizations, and stakeholder networks, and also as key actors influencing each of the building blocks, as health workers, managers and policy-makers.

Different stakeholders may each see the purpose of the system differently (as in Box 2.4), a series of perspectives that can offer new insights into how the health system works, why it has problems, how it can be improved, and how changes made to one component of the system influence the other components (52).

BOX 2.4 SYSTEM STAKEHOLDER NETWORKS

The concept of "multi-finality" shows how stakeholder perspectives on the health system could vary. A health system could be considered:

- a "profit making system" from the perspective of private providers
- a "distribution system" from the perspective of the pharmaceutical industry
- an "employment system" from the perspective of health workers
- a "market system" from the perspective of household consumers and providers of health-related goods and services
- a "health resource system" from the perspective of clients
- a "social support system" from the perspective of local community
- a "complex system" from the perspective of researchers / evaluators
- a set of "policy systems" from the perspective of government
- a set of "sub-systems" from the perspective of the Ministry of Health

Health systems may also be considered by some development aid donors as a "black box" with unacceptably low predictability or a "black hole" where funding goes in, but little comes out.

Modified from Wikipedia: Systems thinking (http://en.wikipedia.org/wiki/Systems_thinking). Accessed October 12, 2009.

BOX 2.5 SYSTEMS THINKING ELEMENTS

Systems organizing	Managing and leading a system; the types of rules that govern the system and set direction through vision and leadership, set prohibitions through regulations and boundary setting, and provide permissions through setting incentives or providing resources
Systems networks	Understanding and managing system stakeholders; the web of all stakeholders and actors, individual and institutional, in the system, through understanding, including, and managing the networks
Systems dynamics	Conceptually modeling and understanding dynamic change; attempting to conceptualize, model and understand dynamic change through analyzing organizational structure and how that influences behaviour of the system
Systems knowledge	Managing content and infrastructure for explicit and tacit knowledge; the critical role of information flows in driving the system towards change, and using the feedback chains of data, information and evidence for guiding decisions

Modified from Best et al, 2007 (22).

Another view of interventions

Health interventions may be aimed at individuals (through clinical or technical interventions such as new drugs, vaccines and diagnostics) or at populations (through public health interventions such as health education or legislative efforts). These interventions often have implications for health systems that are more complicated than first appreciated. When interventions primarily aim to change or strengthen the health system itself, the issue becomes even more complicated with regard to how the system responds. Such interventions are thus inherently more complex to design and evaluate appropriately. Systems thinking looks at a complex intervention as a system in itself, interacting with other building blocks of the system and setting off reactions that may well be unexpected or unpredictable. Apart from a small number of studies, the interaction between health systems and health interventions is not well understood or explored (37). Table 2.2 illustrates some typical system-level interventions.

Systems thinking sees a complex intervention as a system in itself, interacting with other building blocks of the system and setting off reactions that may be unexpected or unpredicted – in the absence of a systems thinking approach

Table 2.2   Typical system-level interventions targeting individual or multiple building blocks

Building block	Common types of interventions
Governance	- Decentralization - Civil society participation - Licensure, accreditation, registration
Financing	- User fees - Conditional cash transfers (demand side) - Pay-for-performance (supply side) - Health insurance - Provider financing modalities - Sector Wide Approaches (SWAps) and basket funding
Human Resources	- Integrated Training - Quality improvement, performance management - Incentives for retention or remote area deployment
Information	- Shifting to electronic (versus manual) medical records - Integrated data systems & enterprise architecture for HIS design - Coordination of national household surveys (e.g. timing of data collected)
Medical products, vaccines and technologies	- New approaches to pharmacovigilance - Supply chain management - Integrated delivery of products and interventions
Service delivery	- Approaches to ensure continuity of care - Integration of services versus centrally managed programmes - Community outreach versus fixed clinics
Multiple building blocks	- Health sector reforms - District health system strengthening

Intervening at high leverage points in the system

A health system, as with any adaptive system, is vulnerable to certain leverage or "tipping" points at which an apparently small intervention can result in substantial system-wide change (53). For instance, a seemingly minor event (e.g. freezing health worker salaries) may tip the system into large-scale change or crisis (e.g. provoking a health worker strike). On the positive side, such interactions could also be managed in a way that leads to synergies. However, it is often difficult to identify such leverage points, and there is no easy formula for finding them. While systems analysis can be instructive as to where such leverage points may be found, more often than not interventions are selected based on intuition and the prevailing development paradigms. A summary of interventions in other (non-health) systems (53), suggests that high leverage points are located in two sub-systems – governance and information. These are two of the health system's building blocks, and the two that receive the least attention from health system interventionists (24). Missing information flows are often identified as the most common cause of system malfunction (43), and incapable or overstretched governance structures can contribute to less than optimal performance and cohesion among the building blocks and for the system as a whole.

Implications of systems thinking for designing and evaluating health interventions

In this chapter we have introduced systems thinking in broad concepts and how this relates to health systems. We have shown how systems thinking takes account of patterns of interaction and patterns of change. Considering and appreciating the intricacies of the health system does not mean adding undue complexity to what appears a simple intervention designed to achieve one outcome. However, it does mean that in designing and evaluating *system-level* interventions or interventions with system-wide effects, a comprehensive assessment of the main effects (intended or not) *and* the contextual factors that may help explain the success or failure of the intervention are essential. This is also instrumental in foreseeing and monitoring consequences, especially negative or unintended, and designing mechanisms to measure and address them (54). Multi-disciplinary and multi-stakeholder involvement is central to this process and cannot be over-emphasized, especially for health systems research (19).

Chapter 3 shows how to develop and evaluate a health system intervention from a systems thinking perspective by using an example to illustrate the full range of ramifications and steps in its practical application.

3

Systems thinking: Applying a systems perspective to design and evaluate health systems interventions

Key messages

- The design and eventual evaluation of any health system intervention must consider its possible effects across all major sub-systems of the health system.

- A collective systems thinking exercise among an inclusive set of health system stakeholders is critical to designing more robust interventions and their evaluations.

- A conceptual pathway of dynamic sub-system interactions can help forecast how the intervention will trigger reactions in the system, and how the system itself will respond.

- Following collective brainstorming and mapping conceptual pathways, interventions may be re-designed to bundle in additional elements amplifying previously unappreciated synergies and mitigating potentially negative effects.

- Probability designs (randomized controlled trials) of large-scale health system interventions are often considered the best designs with high internal validity to evaluate efficacy, but are not always feasible or acceptable; when the are, they are rarely sufficient without complementary contextual and economic evaluations.

- Plausibility designs and other designs that use mixed methods to provide estimates of adequacy, processes, contexts, effects and economic analyses are often the more appropriate design for evaluations of interventions with system-wide effects.

"A systems perspective can minimize the mess; many of today's problems are because of yesterday's solutions"
Dr. Irene Akua Agyepong, Ghana Health Service
Ministry of Health, Ghana, 2009

Introduction

WHO has provided a single people-centered framework combining six clearly defined building blocks or sub-systems that, taken together, comprise a complete health system (20;21). As argued in Chapter 2, understanding the relationships and dynamics among these sub-systems is crucial in the design and evaluation of system-level interventions and interventions with system-wide effects. We must consider both the intervention and the system as complex and dynamic when designing the intervention and its evaluation (17;26;55-58).

This Chapter builds on the definitions and concepts introduced in Chapters 1 and 2, and uses the case of a major contemporary system-level intervention to demonstrate both the systems thinking and the more conventional approaches. The "Ten Steps to Systems Thinking" developed here is intended to provide guidance on applying the systems perspective for a broad audience of designers, implementers, stewards, evaluators and funders. For any intervention with system-wide effects, we ask:

- how can we anticipate potential effects?

- how can we conceptualize the actual behaviour of the intervention? and

- how can we redesign a more sophisticated intervention that accounts for those potential effects?

Answering these questions leads into wider issues of evaluation, and underlines the importance of designing, funding and implementing an evaluation before the intervention is rolled out in order to capture baselines, comparators and the full range of effects over time.

Systems thinking: A case illustration

Performance-based funding (PBF) has emerged in recent years as a popular paradigm both in developed countries and for development assistance. In the health sector, two specific instruments of performance-based funding are attracting attention of countries and donors seeking to boost performance in health systems. These are paying-for-performance (P4P) and conditional cash transfers (CCTs) (59-63). Paying-for-performance is usually implemented as a supply-side cash incentive given to health care providers on achievement of a pre-specified performance target. Conditional cash transfers are a demand-side cash incentive given to clients of the health system to encourage them to adopt particular health behaviours or utilize a specified health service. They are both system-level interventions that target multiple building blocks (service delivery and financing), with potentially powerful effects on other sub-systems.

As these major system-level interventions are extended to a national scale, health system stakeholders need to know whether they work, for whom they work, and under what particular conditions and contexts. All too often they must do this without the benefit of small-scale pilot studies, as these may be politically difficult or operationally meaningless. For a P4P intervention that puts a cash bonus in the pockets of health workers, stakeholders will need to know if the intervention is good value for money – money that might otherwise be invested directly in improving health services or other aspects of the system.

Anticipating relationships and reactions among the sub-systems and the various actors in the system is essential in predicting possible system-wide implications and effects.

BOX 3.1 A PAY-FOR-PERFORMANCE INTERVENTION - AN ILLUSTRATIVE EXAMPLE[1]

In a low-income country, the Ministry of Health, Ministry of Finance and their international funding partners decide to launch a Pay-for-Performance (P4P) programme to improve service quality. After internal discussion, they determine that tuberculosis care and treatment is unacceptably weak, and that a P4P programme could be used to increase the effective coverage of Tuberculosis Directly Observed Short Course Treatment (TB DOTS). The P4P intervention specifies that cash awards will be paid to TB DOTS health care providers every six months upon successful achievement of targets for increased coverage (utilization and adherence) rates. Every health facility in the country negotiates their own effective coverage targets, and the country's health information system (HIS) will be used to monitor the targets.

The Problem: low rates of TB patient uptake and adherence to TB DOTS in detected cases.

The Policy Response: introduction of financial incentives for TB DOTS providers who succeed in increasing uptake and adherence rates.

Anticipated Outputs: incremental improvements in uptake and adherence rates.

Results: adherence rates increase by x%. Costs of the incentive package increase by y%.

Anticipated Outcomes: higher effectiveness of TB DOTS in reducing morbidity, mortality and risk of TB.

Following two years of implementation, the official evaluation of the programme focused on costs to the health system and TB DOTS adherence rates. It concluded that the programme was a success. However, though not part of the official evaluation, some field-based staff reported fundamental problems with the programme. They observed that health facility staff were moving towards the more "lucrative" TB services at the expense of other core services, compromising the quality of services each facility offered. Some reported widespread gaming and even outright corruption, which the weak HIS was unable to capture.

While these issues may have remained an unavoidable but manageable consequence of improved TB services, a sudden measles epidemic brought all of these problems into new light. With fewer capable staff at most health facilities, the system was less able to manage cases or prevent the epidemic from spreading. Many observers increasingly felt that the benefits of the TB programme were more than offset by the increased costs, morbidity and mortality elsewhere in the health system.

Could these problems have been identified and mitigated at the design stage of the intervention?

---

[1] This case illustration is a hypothetical example composed of experiences from a number of real cases.

The more conventional approach to the intervention. As a pay-for-performance instrument, the goal of a P4P is to achieve an impact on a specific issue. In essence, the P4P "purchases" and supports a narrow component of health care delivery. Without a systems perspective, interest tends to centre on this narrow component, and the linear process, output, outcome and eventual impact of the investment. Notably, the intervention funder itself typically contracts the evaluation of the P4P and the target disease programme, and sets the parameters they want evaluated. The resultant evaluation only illuminates the most obvious direct, linear inputs and expected effects of the intervention in terms of costs, coverage, uptake and equity of the intervention in question.

Figure 3.1 illustrates the more conventional approach. The P4P intervention targets service delivery through increased financing, and operates on the assumption that health workers will change something in the quality of TB DOTs

service delivery to improve patient uptake and adherence. This will likely manifest itself in local low- or no-cost innovations in attracting patients to diagnosis, and maintaining them on treatment. The assumption here is that improved quality translates to more effective coverage, which in turn results in better health in the population, and better equity and responsiveness of the health system itself.

Revisiting the intervention from a systems perspective. Since the P4P is a major, high-cost, system-level intervention operating through a new financing mechanism, it demands a systems perspective (29;33;64), including fuller use of system leadership and broader networks (stakeholders), systems organization, and systems knowledge (see Chapter 2 for a discussion of these concepts) (22). In moving beyond the "input-blackbox-output" paradigm, the systems perspective considers inputs, outputs, initial, intermediate and eventual outcomes, *and* feedback, processes, flows, control and contexts (22).

In the more conventional approach, interest is centered on the linear process, output, outcome and eventual impact of the intervention.

In moving beyond the "input-blackbox-output" paradigm, the systems perspective considers inputs, outputs, initial, intermediate and eventual outcomes, and feedback, processes, flows, control and contexts.

Figure 3.1 More conventional pathway from P4P financing intervention to expected effects

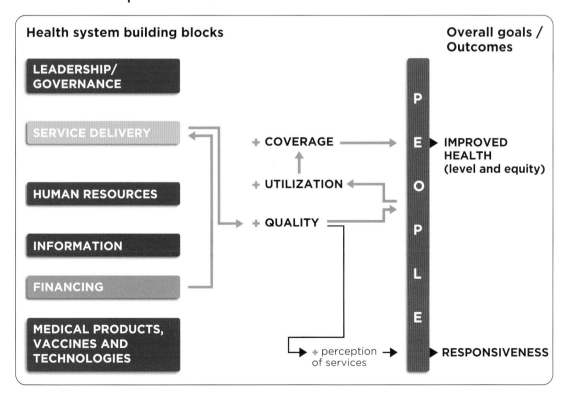

Ten Steps to Systems Thinking

As a guide to applying this perspective, we propose "Ten Steps to Systems Thinking," and use our case illustration to show how they might work in practice. These steps are less an exact and rigid blueprint and more a conceptualized process. They are flexible and may be adapted to many different situations and possibilities.

BOX 3.2 TEN STEPS TO SYSTEMS THINKING: APPLYING A SYSTEMS PERSPECTIVE IN THE DESIGN AND EVALUATION OF INTERVENTIONS

I: Intervention Design

1. **Convene stakeholders:** Identify and convene stakeholders representing each building block, plus selected intervention designers and implementers, users of the health system, and representatives of the research community

2. **Collectively brainstorm:** Collectively deliberate on possible system wide effects of the proposed intervention respecting systems characteristics (feedback, time delays, policy resistance, etc.) and systems dynamics

3. **Conceptualize effects:** Develop a conceptual pathway mapping how the intervention will affect health and the health system through its sub-systems

4. **Adapt and redesign:** Adapt and redesign the proposed intervention to optimize synergies and other positive effects while avoiding or minimizing any potentially major negative effects.

II: Evaluation Design

5. **Determine indicators:** Decide on indicators that are important to track in the re-designed intervention (from process to issues to context) across the affected sub-systems

6. **Choose methods:** Decide on evaluation methods to best track the indicators

7. **Select design:** Opt for the evaluation design that best manages the methods and fits the nature of the intervention

8. **Develop plan and timeline:** Collectively develop an evaluation plan and timeline by engaging the necessary disciplines

9. **Set a budget:** Determine the budget and scale by considering implications for both the intervention and the evaluation partnership

10. **Source funding:** Assemble funding to support the evaluation *before* the intervention begins.

Part I: The Intervention Design

Step 1. Convene stakeholders: Multidisciplinary and multi-stakeholder involvement is a crucial element throughout the "Ten Steps to Systems Thinking" – identifying and convening key stakeholders concerned with or affected by the intervention's implementation is essential. To legitimate the convening process, this should either start with or be endorsed at a high official level in the Ministry of Health. There are a number of approaches for identifying stakeholders (including context mapping and stakeholder analysis) (65;66), however common sense should prevail and err on the side of inclusivity. At a minimum, at least one knowledgeable representative of each sub-system (or building block) is required, plus at least one representative of the research community and one from a funding partner. Not all interventions will need all of the stakeholders described here, however a complex intervention will require increasing levels of consultation.

Step 2. Collectively brainstorm: This step is critical in identifying all possible system-wide effects of the proposed intervention. Once the right mix of stakeholders has convened to discuss the proposed intervention, they anticipate and hypothesize all possible ramifications of the intervention within each building block, while also thinking through the many interactions among the sub-systems. Front-line implementers (possibly those representing the service delivery and health workforce building blocks) will identify potential effects of the implementation pathway. The final aspect of this step will be nominating leaders and a smaller design team to take ownership of the intervention, particularly in conceptualizing its effects, redesigning it, and identifying individuals to develop its evaluation.

BOX 3.3 THE P4P INTERVENTION – CONVENING STAKEHOLDERS

Following official decisions to proceed with the intervention, the Ministry of Health's TB Control Programme Manager requests the Ministry's Chief Medical Officer to convene other concerned directors in the MoH to discuss the opportunity and to identify further stakeholders. This group (representing governance, financing, human resources, information, essential drugs, and service delivery) identifies a range of other stakeholders drawn from representatives of the research community, civil society, the civil service commission, front-line TB DOTs health workers, District Health Management Teams and the funding partner. Following this identification, the Chief Medical Officer organizes a schedule of small, short stakeholder consultations and issues invitations, with the MoH Director of Planning and Policy appointed to facilitate the meetings.

BOX 3.4 THE P4P INTERVENTION – BRAINSTORMING

Under the facilitation of the Director of Policy and Planning, initial stakeholder workshops reveal that the principal potential effects of the P4P intervention on the **service delivery** sub-system may include the improved attractiveness of services due to better access and opening hours, and a more welcoming demeanor and behaviour from health workers. These positive effects should result in increased utilization and hence coverage. However, potentially negative effects may arise if health workers neglect services that are not rewarded by the P4P (crowding out). High-performing health workers may already be more available in advantaged areas than in poorer areas and bonuses may concentrate in their hands, further increasing existing inequities among the served populations. On the other hand, equity might be improved if the P4P attracts workers to disadvantaged areas where the opportunities to improve coverage are perceived as higher, and thus bonuses easier to gain.

The intervention may improve the **information** sub-system to monitor coverage as a key means of assessing whether a bonus should be paid or not. However, given existing weaknesses in the health information system, actors may manipulate it to over-report improvements to receive bonuses without conditional levels actually achieved. The information system may not be capable of providing sufficiently sensitive estimates of the conditional indicator (in this case effective coverage of TB DOTs), and may need direct strengthening to support the P4P.

Potential positive effects on the **human resources** sub-system might be improved provider motivation, including a willingness to work in remote areas. Conversely, intrinsic motivation might be eroded to the point where workers focus exclusively on tasks where additional bonuses can be most easily acquired. Staff conflicts and rivalry may arise among the team and supervisors if only some members qualify for the bonus and if it is unclear how targets for payment are set and monitored. Additionally, there may be trade union or civil service impediments to this sort of employee compensation.

The role of those supply- and demand-side effects depends on a variety of **governance** factors that may change over time, including increased trust and more effective decentralization and ownership. Challenges in meeting public accountability and transparency for the bonus payments may arise. New modalities for handling discretionary cash payments for staff in health facilities may be needed.

Finally, for the **financing** sub-system, there might be incrementally more funding, but also an increased fragmentation of funding modalities – potentially running counter to sector-wide and budget support principles. The management of cash payments to health facilities has both financing and governance implications.

Based on the outcomes of this brainstorming process, the stakeholders then prioritize potential effects according to their importance and likelihood in a tabular format (see Table 3.1) as a basis for a conceptual framework (see Figure 3.2).

Table 3.1 Prioritized potential system-wide effects of the P4P intervention

Priority 1=high 5=low	Effect	Positive + or Negative –	Likelihood (high, medium, low)	Importance (high, medium, low)	Sub-system
1	Staff conflicts if bonus not universal	–	High	High	HR
1	Over-reported improvements	–	High	High	Information
1	Local incentives to seek solutions to delivery issues	+	High	High	Service delivery
2	Resource allocation imbalance (fragmented funding modalities)	–	High	Medium	Financing
2	Difficulties managing cash payments	–	High	Medium	Financing
2	Increased utilization of TB DOTS	+	Medium	High	Service delivery
2	Crowding out of non-target health services	–	Medium	High	Service delivery
2	Frustrated demand for better service infrastructure	–	Medium	High	Service delivery
2	Frustration among public, health workers of increased demand without increased technical quality/quantity	–	Medium	High	Medicines & Technoligies
3	Reduced accountability and transparency regarding bonus payments	–	Medium	Medium	Governance
4	Increased production, use of information/feedback	+	Low	Medium	Information
5	Decentralization (local ownership and control)	+	Low	Low	Governance
5	Reveal and resolve phantom worker issues	+	Low	Low	Governance
5	Increased health worker motivation	+	Low	Low	HR
5	Health worker willingness to accept postings to remote/disadvantaged areas	+	Low	Low	HR
5	Deflection of qualified staff to the level where bonus is achievable	–	Low	Low	HR

Note: this table and Table 3.2 were created at an actual role-playing simulation brainstorming session.

Step 3. Conceptualize effects: In anticipating possible positive and negative effects in the other health sub-systems, it is clear that any major intervention could have important unknowns. In this step, a smaller design team takes the tabular output and develops a conceptual pathway mapping how the intervention will affect health and the health system through its sub-systems, with particular attention to feedback loops. This conceptual pathway of dynamic interactions shows how the intervention will trigger reactions in the system, and how the system might respond (38;67). This highlights key potential negative and positive effects at all major sub-systems in the health systems framework. While this is an initial pathway, evaluation designs will need to consider that interventions will play out differently in different settings with different actors. Concept mapping (68) and systems dynamic modeling (33) are possible tools to use at this stage (see Chapter 4 for a discussion of concept mapping).

A conceptual pathway of dynamic interactions shows how the intervention will trigger reactions in the system, and how the system might respond

Step 4. Adapt and redesign: In this final design step, the initial concept for the intervention will likely need to be adapted or re-designed in light of the first three steps to optimize synergies and other positive effects while avoiding or minimizing any potentially major negative effects. Based on the expected or hypothesized causal pathway of dynamic interactions from Step 3 and the table of potential effects brainstormed in Step 2, the stakeholders may re-think their intervention design to bundle in additional design elements to mitigate important negative effects, maximize previously unappreciated potential synergies or avoid any possible obstacles. This is a collective exercise in prioritizing the negative effects into those that are potentially serious, and determining whether and how to amplify the positive effects. The group's response to these effects will contribute directly to ideas for the adaptation or redesign of the intervention.

Figure 3.2 Conceptual pathway for the P4P intervention using a systems perspective

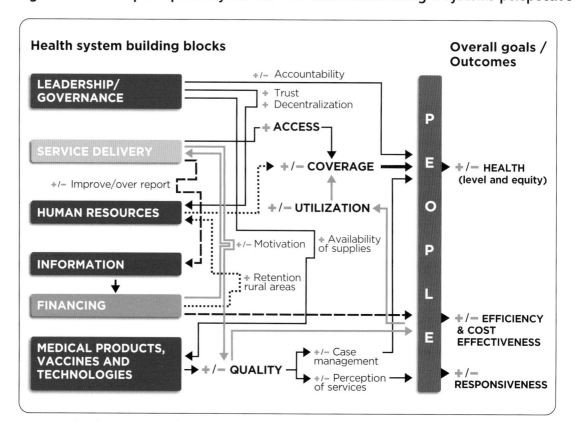

BOX 3.5 THE P4P INTERVENTION – REDESIGN

In the P4P example, the design team advocates for additional complementary funding to strengthen the health information system to improve the statistics used to trigger the pay-for-performance bonus. They restructure how bonuses are awarded across all staff of the facility, and the district or regional authorities who support those facilities. They also decide to bundle or raise additional support to handle the anticipated increased demand for health services, and spread the P4P over a broader spectrum of essential services to avoid crowding out. Lastly, they recommend opening bank accounts for health facilities to manage timely disbursement of bonuses.

While led by the design team that conceptualized the effects in Step 3, the product created in Step 4 – the adapted design for the intervention – will ideally be returned to the larger stakeholder group. This group may elect to convene again, and may engage in further brainstorming to consider and weigh the innovations added at this stage.

Once the intervention design has been finalized, the stakeholders need to decide how it should be expanded nation-wide, and begin to consider the evaluation design. Below, in Part II of this Chapter, we consider each of the steps in the evaluation design. The discussion is targeted in particular at researchers and evaluators.

Figure 3.3 Major moments in Steps 1 – 5

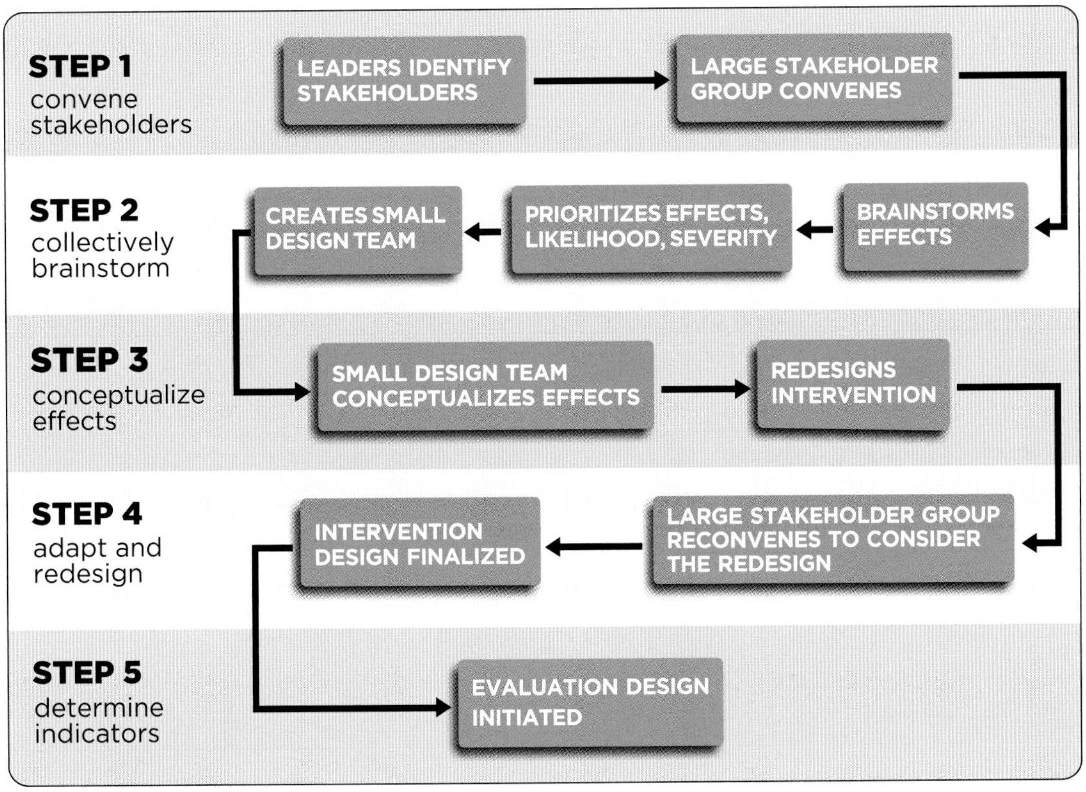

Part II: The evaluation design

Step 5. Determine indicators: Once the intervention has been designed or re-designed using the systems perspective, the design team, now assisted by researchers and/or evaluators, need to develop the key research questions to inform the evaluation. They must decide what processes, issues and contexts are important to track over time in the evaluation, considering the major positive and negative effects hypothesized and discussed during steps 1-4. Once the research questions have been agreed upon, the next issue is to decide upon necessary indicators, and the potential data sources for these indicators. Table 3.2 (following Step 6) shows indicators, data sources and evaluation types for the P4P case illustration.

Step 6. Choose methods: Once the indicators and potential data sources have been agreed upon, the next decision is selecting the best methods to generate the required data.

To deal with the complexity of large-scale system-level interventions, the evaluation should include four components: a **process evaluation** (for adequacy); a **context evaluation** (for transferability); an **effects evaluation** (to gauge the intervention's effects across all sub-systems); and an **economic evaluation** (to determine value for money). This requires baseline, formative (during early implementation) and summative (during advanced implementation) evaluations, with special attention during the formative evaluation phase to generate lessons in order to fine-tune the intervention – to improve performance and to understand how the intervention really works given the characteristics of systems (see Figure 3.4).

The **process evaluation** component addresses adequacy and helps explain: what processes of change lead to observed effects; why outcomes might not have changed; and if the intervention is working as expected within and across the sub-systems. For instance, the process evaluation could address the governance sub-system in terms of looking at policy formulation, programme acceptability among stakeholders, priority setting at various levels, and guideline availability. It could address the financing sub-system by examining financial flows, sustainability and (re)allocations of additional funds to scale-up technologies, infrastructure and supplies in the system. For the human resources sub-system, the training and availability of guidelines, the extent of training coverage and actual financing could all serve as indicators to track the degree of implementation. For the other sub-systems, the process evaluation could focus on the process of implementation and how this affects different aspects of service delivery over time – including provider motivation, technical and human quality of care.

The **context evaluation** component can help explain whether the observed effects are due to the intervention – and if not, why not? – essential to ensuring the plausibility of the evaluation's conclusions. The importance of context within the system can never be over-estimated since the personal and institutional contexts shape the behaviours of the actors as much as the structural context of the system. This requires ruling out the influence of external factors and bringing into play the importance of comparison areas and adjusting for confounders (69). A context evaluation is also essential for the eventual transferability of the results by documenting circumstances in which the intervention operated, what effects the intervention in this context produced, and for whom the effects were observed (17).

The **effects evaluation** component is the one most commonly conducted and understood and needs little elaboration here. It basically describes and quantifies the intervention's health outcomes as well as its impact on effective coverage, quality of care, and equity – issues that correspond with the overall goals/outcomes of the health system.

The **economic evaluation** component measures the intervention's cost-effectiveness by looking at incremental costs of implementing the intervention from the provider and wider societal perspectives (including the perspective of households) compared with the status quo or other alternatives. It thus addresses efficiency concerns, one of the overall outcomes of the health system framework (26;70). It can also include a financial assessment of the programme's sustainability, and comparison of its cost per capita to other services.

Figure 3.4 Key components and generic research questions for evaluations

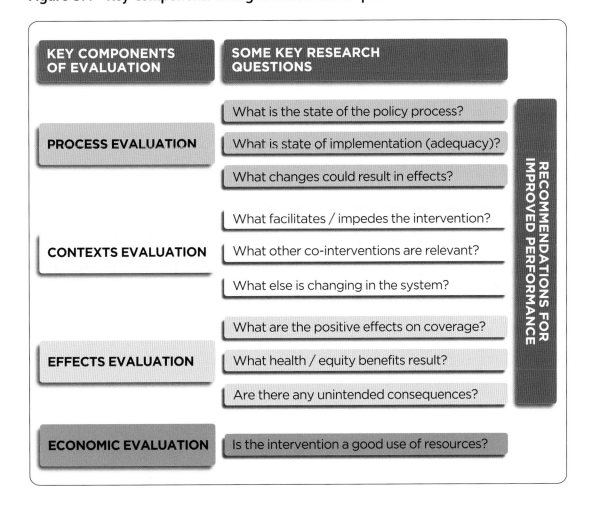

Table 3.2 A selection of research questions, indicators and data sources for the P4P intervention

Type of evaluation	Key research questions	Quantitative indicators	Qualitative indicators	Data Source
Process	Is P4P being implemented as intended?	■ Availability of implementation guidelines at appropriate levels of the health system ■ Proportion of stakeholders who have received training on P4P at appropriate levels of the health system ■ Time between submission of six monthly reports and payment of bonuses ■ How much bonus do health facilities and health workers get, by cadre ■ Quantity of bonus payments made to health facilities ■ Extent of system leakage; frequency of receipt of bonus by non-eligible facilities or staff ■ Frequency of managerial identification of mis-reporting of performance	■ Method of allocating bonus payments within a health facility ■ Who receives bonus payments ■ Punitive methods, if any, for dealing with misreported indicators when identified by management	■ In-depth interviews and FGDs ■ Health facility survey ■ In-depth interviews and FGDs ■ Health facility survey ■ Exit interviews
Contexts	What other financing or human resource interventions are underway during the P4P extension?	■ Training coverage	■ Type of trainings	■ Document review ■ FGDs

Type of evaluation	Key research questions	Quantitative indicators	Qualitative indicators	Data Source
Contexts	What other service delivery interventions targeting maternal and neonatal interventions are underway during the F4P extension?	■ Training coverage	■ Type of trainings	■ Document review ■ FGDs
	What other service delivery interventions are made for non-target services?	■ Training coverage	■ Type of trainings	■ Document review ■ FGDs
	What measures have been taken to improve health information systems and their audits?		■ Changes made	■ In-depth interviews ■ Document reviews
	What other changes in society may effect access and utilization of health services?		■ Factors affecting access to concerned health facilities, e.g. economic, availability of public transport ■ Location of health facilities, compared to other types of providers	■ Secondary document review (e.g. household budget surveys, district records, etc.)

Type of evaluation	Key research questions	Quantitative indicators	Qualitative indicators	Data Source
Effects	What is the effect of P4P on provider motivation and trust relations?	■ Some quantitative measures of motivation	■ Perceived impact of P4P on provider motivation over time ■ Possible variations in perceptions of key stakeholders about the adequacy of the bonus level over time ■ Impact of P4P on trust between stakeholders	■ In-depth interviews and FGDs ■ Health facility survey
	What is the effect of P4P on resource allocation?	■ Amount of funds available at facility level and patterns of expenditure within facilities	■ Method of budget allocation and priority investments at district level	■ In-depth interviews and FGDs ■ Document review
	What is the effect of P4P on service quality and availability?	■ Average consultation duration in minutes for targeted and non-targeted services before and after intervention ■ Proportion of patients receiving drugs or treatments at health facility for targeted and non-targeted services ■ Rates of referral for delivery care ■ Structural quality score ■ Time spent by health workers on activities associated with bonus payment, vs. activities with no associated bonus ■ Total number of health workers in facility	■ Patient satisfaction with targeted and non-targeted services ■ Patient reports on costs of services	■ Health facility survey ■ Household survey ■ Exit interviews ■ Time motion study

Type of evaluation	Key research questions	Quantitative indicators	Qualitative indicators	Data Source
		■ User charges for targeted and non-targeted services		
Effects	What is the effect of P4P on coverage?	■ Coverage rates of services linked to bonus payment (including c-section proportions) by socio-economic status ■ Coverage rates of non-targeted services (including ante-natal care, family planning, and total out- and in-patient admissions)	■ Willingness of staff to move to under-staffed, more remote facilities as a result of the P4P scheme (ideally by identifying staff who have actually moved for this reason).	■ HMIS ■ Health facility survey – record review ■ Household survey ■ Document review
Economic	Is P4P cost-effective? Is P4P affordable? What is the optimal P4P bonus level?	■ Overall economic status of target population of facilities receiving higher level bonus payments and those receiving lower levels, or not receiving bonus payments ■ P4P as proportion of provider income ■ Effect of P4P on proportional spending in overall health budget ■ Incremental cost-effectiveness of P4P compared to other measures of improving quality of care or increasing coverage, or even wider range of interventions ■ Cost per additional coverage ■ Cost per capita		■ Financial accounts for P4P and comparator intervention ■ District budget per capita for different services ■ Document review ■ Household survey

Step 7. Select design: There are some evaluation designs particularly well-suited to system-level interventions. These tend to come more from the epidemiologic and health systems research tradition than from the monitoring and evaluation tradition. In this step, we discuss the most common designs – probability designs, plausibility designs, and adequacy designs.

Probability designs. Purely experimental methods – randomized controlled trials (RCTs) – are considered the "gold standard" for evaluations in health research and have been used primarily in the evaluation of intervention efficacy and occasionally for health systems strengthening interventions. However, RCTs tend to be carried out in limited areas and over a relatively short period of time, making them often ill-suited to evaluating interventions with system-wide effects, especially those with long delays in expected effects or where causality is complex and difficult to establish. Probability designs are thus not often an ideal approach to evaluation using the systems perspective.

BOX 3.6 THE P4P INTERVENTION – PROBABILITY DESIGN

The evaluators felt it might be possible to apply a cluster randomized controlled design for evaluation, depending on how the intervention is actually implemented at scale (33;70-72). Such a design would work if, for example, it were politically acceptable to randomly assign a set of intervention areas (e.g. districts) – each would introduce identical financial performance contracts, with a control group composed of areas not receiving the intervention.

As observed above, however, randomization alone will not illuminate the complex causal pathway between intervention and sub-systems; will not easily allow for delays in effects or changes over time in contextual factor; and is further weakened by the constant reform of health systems typically subject to a variety of interventions in multiple sub-systems at the same time. RCTs alone simply lack the operational plausibility and generalizability to other contexts unless special attention is paid to documenting contexts (51).

Partly for the above reasons, purely experimental randomized controlled trials of health systems interventions are not common (73). While there are examples where RCTs have been successfully used to evaluate such interventions at scale (74), in many circumstances, they are simply inappropriate, inadequate, possibly unethical or impossible to conduct (75)

In large-scale system-level interventions, a phased introduction is typical. Interventions rolled out nation-wide cannot be launched everywhere simultaneously and often take one or several years to reach all administrative areas of a country. It may then be possible to use a randomized step-wedge design. In a step-wedge design, an intervention is sequentially expanded to administrative regions over a number of time periods. Ideally, the order in which the different geographic administrative areas receive the intervention is determined at random and, by the end of the random allocation, all areas will have received the intervention. Step-wedge designs offer a number of opportunities for data analysis, as well as for modeling the element of time on the effectiveness of an intervention. However there are very few examples of step-wedge designs applied to the evaluation of a system-level intervention (76).

Given these very real limitations, most system-level interventions usually roll-out in a non-random manner – often in the easiest-to-reach areas first and then progressing to more difficult areas, making time series and equity effects more difficult to interpret. There is also a learning and maturation phenomenon that changes the intervention over time in such real-world implementation. It has been shown that this non-random extension can result in completely different conclusions, for example, on equity during the early, mid- and late phases of the roll-out (Box 3.1; Figure 3.5).

Plausibility designs. In recognition of these constraints on RCTs, plausibility designs have emerged as the most suitable substitute for evaluating the effectiveness of complex, large-scale, system-level interventions in real-life settings. Plausibility designs demonstrate that a specific intervention, when adequately delivered, is effective in its context (69;77;77-80). They often include descriptive studies on the adequacy of the intervention's delivery (are expected processes taking place?) but then go beyond with additional observational studies (are the observed changes plausibly due to the adequacy of the expected processes?).

Plausibility designs require comprehensive documentation of contexts to exclude external factors as the explanation for observed changes; they also need a comparison area or group that allows adjustment for confounding factors and identification of contextual factors critical to an intervention's success (or failure) alongside conceptual frameworks for how the intervention is expected to have an effect. Even in situations where there is convincing evidence from RCTs at the initial phase of an intervention's development, it is important to do plausibility designs over the long term when the intervention is rolled out under conditions closer to routine. Such designs are most useful when there are relatively rapid and widespread effects in large populations; where confounding is unlikely to explain observed effects; where selection bias is unlikely; and where there are objective measures of exposure. Even when effects are widespread, results should still be interpreted cautiously, especially if those effects are unexpected. Plausibility designs are in a sense both observational and analytical.

Adequacy designs. Adequacy designs are important for complex interventions that consist of a suite of associated activities or interventions, and are usually included in plausibility designs. These designs may be useful for policy-makers when there is no improvement in the outcome of interest, or where there is a large improvement in a relatively simple outcome combined with a relatively short causal chain, and where confounding is unlikely. Although many system-level interventions have long causal chains and delays in effect, adequacy designs, although necessary, are rarely sufficient on their own. They are descriptive and do not allow for control of confounders.

BOX 3.7 THE P4P INTERVENTION – EVALUATION TYPE

Given this consideration of three different designs, the design team determine that a plausibility design is the most practical option for the evaluation of the P4P intervention.

Table 3.3 Summary of characteristics for optional evaluation design choices for the P4P intervention

Design	Characteristics	Advantages	Disadvantages
Probability	Cluster (district) randomized controlled trial (RCT) design applied to all components of the intervention	▪ Controls for confounders ▪ Generates strong evidence of efficacy ▪ Probability of confounding can be estimated	▪ Delays full implementation ▪ Does not explain causal link between intervention and outcomes ▪ Misrepresents dynamic properties of the system ▪ Fails to take account of contextual and emergent aspects ▪ Challenge for health system policies acting at district level or higher ▪ Political acceptability difficult
	Cluster randomized controlled design applied to individual components of the intervention (e.g. P4P with and without performance contracts)	▪ May be politically more acceptable as all areas receive the same funding	▪ Cannot control for effects of cash payments *per se* except through before-after study
	Randomized step-wedge controlled trial	▪ May be more politically acceptable in terms of roll-out	▪ As with all RCTs, contextual documentation needs to be added
Plausibility	Internal comparison (e.g. early and late starter districts)	▪ Controls for most confounders ▪ All plausibility designs include measures of adequacy and context	▪ Difficulty controlling for inherent differences between early starters and late starters ▪ Relies on natural phasing-in
	External comparison (e.g. comparison districts)	▪ May be more acceptable than randomization	▪ Need to control for confounding or inherent differences between intervention and comparison areas
	Interrupted time-series	▪ Allows evaluator to control for the natural trend that would have occurred anyway, in the outcome indicators	▪ Requires reliable data on core indicators up to a year before the start of the intervention, to allow for trend estimation
Adequacy	Historical comparison (before and after study)	▪ Does not require political "buy in"	▪ Can only control qualitatively for confounders, hence assessment of effects is less robust. Absence of baseline in midstream evaluation is often a problem

Step 8. Develop plan and timeline: Once decisions on the research questions, indicators, data sources, methodological approach and type of design have been made, it is then possible to identify the necessary disciplines and expand the partners required to complete the evaluation plan.

Timing of evaluations. The pace at which health system strengthening investments and innovations occur is quickening. Most often, system-level interventions are planned, funded, and launched before its accompanying evaluation can be properly commissioned, designed and funded. The majority of evaluations, if done, have no **baseline evaluation** because the evaluations often start mid-stream, long after the intervention has been rolled out. An additional timing weakness occurs when evaluations do not run long enough to detect indirect or long-term effects that often take time to develop.

Evaluation plan. There is also a need after the **baseline evaluation** to include a **formative evaluation** in the intervention's early stages (to fine-tune the intervention and adapt its implementation). To some extent then, the formative evaluation becomes part of the intervention, and makes the **impact evaluation** more complex. But this is relevant because of the potential for variation in implementation in complex systems in different settings. Finally, since complex, system-level interventions will be variously implemented or experienced in different facilities or areas, the impact evaluation should deliberately estimate how its effects vary across sites or areas – what the maximum and minimum effects are – rather than just focusing on the average effect (which might hide different experiences). This would allow for richer discussion of replicability in other settings – e.g. when the intervention is rolled out in other parts of the country – and offer some guidance on how to support interventions elsewhere.

BOX 3.8 NON-RANDOM ROLL-OUT OF INTERVENTIONS AND THE TIMING OF EVALUATIONS

The Tanzania National Voucher Scheme (TNVS) is a national programme delivering vouchers for subsidised insecticide-treated nets to women at antenatal clinics. It was scaled up gradually over the period of about 18 months starting in October 2004.

The evaluation of the TNVS was designed to capture both the levels of coverage achieved by the voucher scheme, and its socioeconomic distribution (80). For the evaluation, districts were classified into three equal-sized groups, according to their planned launch date, and a random sample of seven districts from each of these three strata was selected. Household, facility and facility user surveys were conducted in the 21 evaluation districts (81) and socioeconomic status of beneficiaries was measured using a combination of household asset ownership and housing conditions, and a single asset index was estimated for the whole sample. Households were divided into quintiles according to their value of the continuous SES index estimated using principal components analysis over the whole sample of districts.

This SES analysis allowed evaluation of the socioeconomic distribution of households according to the programme launch date – "early," "middle" and "late". The predominance of poorest (Q1) in the "late" launch group, and the least poor (Q5) in the "early" launch districts shows how the non-random roll-out plan favoured the least poor parts of the country first. The extended roll-out period, probably essential in a country the size of Tanzania, means that many of the poorest districts and households received the intervention up to 18 months later than the first ones. This evidence about roll out and SES also demonstrates the challenge of programme evaluation when scale up is non-random: programme exposure is positively correlated with socioeconomic status, making it important to control for this factor when undertaking analysis of programme impact and sustaining the evaluation long enough to make valid conclusions (80).

Source: Text provided by Hanson K, Marchant T, Nathan R, Bruce J, Mponda H, Jones C. and Lengeler, C, and presented in part at the Swiss Tropical Institute *Symposium on Health System Strengthening: Role of conditional cash incentives?* November 27, 2008, Basel, Switzerland.

Figure 3.5 Socioeconomic distribution of households by launch of insecticide-treated nets (ITNs) voucher scheme in the United Republic of Tanzania

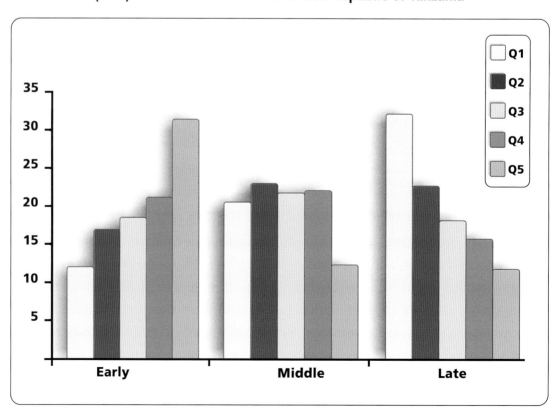

Step 9. Set a budget: This step can sometimes be part of step 8, but in a competitive grants process it may not be possible to know the cost implications of the evaluation until step 8 is completed. Ideally the evaluation budget should revert to the design group for inclusion with the intervention budget. This will ensure the funding is in place before the intervention is implemented.

Step 10. Source funding: The last step is to encourage an evaluation that is front-loaded and funded before the intervention commences its roll out in order to provide the counterfactual baselines for all measures. One consequence of the improved intervention design and improved evaluation design is the likely higher cost for both (but higher probability of successful implementation and accurate evaluation).

Conclusion

This chapter provides further detail on how a systems perspective can create a more dynamic design and evaluation of a system-level intervention intending to strengthen the health system. The Ten Steps to Systems Thinking demonstrate practically how to link the acts of planning, design and evaluation in a more coherent, participatory and system-centred way.

Beyond the importance of the intervention design, this Chapter calls particular attention to the centrality of evaluation in documenting and assessing effects. Ideally, evaluations should be designed, funded and started before the intervention is rolled out in order to provide adequate baselines and comparators. This is essential if we are to fully demonstrate the effectiveness of the intervention and its system-wide impacts. Intervention and evaluation funders should be prepared for the higher costs of comprehensive evaluations addressing the broader effects of health system strengthening. Evaluations that fail to capture and assess the full systemic effects of an intervention may be highly misleading. The systems perspective will reward its funders and designers with a comprehensive assessment of whether the intervention works, how, for whom, and under what circumstances.

4

Systems thinking for health systems: Challenges and opportunities in real-world settings

Key messages

- With leadership, conviction and commitment, systems thinking can open powerful pathways to identify and resolve health system challenges.

- Health system stewards can use the systems thinking perspective to increase local ownership of multi-stakeholder processes and respond to the dynamic of disease-specific, sometimes donor-driven "solutions".

- Engaging "street-level" policy implementers at the design stage of new interventions can enhance ownership of the intervention and increase the potential for its successful implementation.

- Strengthening the governance and leadership roles of health systems stewards is a crucial step in strengthening health systems.

> *"The first of the 'fundamental impediments' to the adoption of systems thinking is that we're prisoners of our frame of reference"*
> Barry Richmond, 1991 (82)

Introduction

Previous Chapters of this Report have emphasized the valuable contributions of systems thinking in designing and evaluating interventions to strengthen health systems. Although the rationale and potential for applying the systems perspective in public health are not new (22;29;34-37), many practitioners still tend to dismiss it as too complicated or unsuited for any practical purpose or application (22).

Following Chapter 2's broad overview of systems thinking, and the "Ten Steps to Systems Thinking" illustrated in Chapter 3, this Chapter discusses systems thinking in the real world – where the pressures and dynamics of actual situations often block or blur the systems perspective. Systems thinking must resonate with existing experiences in developing countries and account for present challenges in its application and integration. For those who wish to improve present realities and relationships using the systems perspective – from researchers to system stewards to international funders – this Chapter underlines how systems thinking can identify and resolve various health system challenges, and highlights some particularly innovative approaches and experiences.

Part I: Select challenges in applying a systems perspective

There are a host of challenges to applying a systems perspective in developing countries, ranging from prevailing development paradigms to issues around intervention implementation.

In this Chapter, we do not propose systems thinking as a panacea to resolve or restructure the relationships at the heart of a health system; rather, we use it as a tool to identify where some of the key blockages and challenges in strengthening health systems lie. Beyond the overarching resistance to systems thinking – and how it might upset the relationships that fund and support the dominant approaches to improving health – we identify four specific challenges in applying a systems perspective, and suggest how this perspective can convert them into opportunities to strengthen health systems.

Many still tend to dismiss systems thinking as too complicated for any practical purpose or application.

BOX 4.1 SELECT CHALLENGES IN APPLYING A SYSTEMS PERSPECTIVE

- Aligning policies, priorities and perspectives among donors and national policy-makers

- Managing and coordinating partnerships and expectations among system stakeholders

- Implementing and fostering ownership of interventions at the national and sub-national level

- Building capacity at the country level to apply a systems analytic perspective

---

BOX 4.2 DEFINING HEALTH SYSTEMS STEWARDS

In this Chapter we focus on national health system stewards, which we understand as policy-makers and leaders responsible for providing strategic direction to the system and its concerned stakeholders. These are typically from government (e.g. senior Ministry of Health officials, a district commissioner, a hospital administrator), but may also include other stakeholders, e.g. civil society and the private sector. System stewards are "information providers and change agents, linking the general public, consumer groups, civic society, the research community, professional organizations and the government in improving health of the people in a participatory way"(83).

1. Aligning policies, priorities and perspectives among donors and national policy-makers

"HIV, TB and Malaria have taken almost 90% of our time, not to mention that they have also taken most of our budgetary money to the extent that we have actually neglected what we call non-communicable diseases"
Ministry of Health official, Zambia,
October 2007 (84).

There is a tension in many developing country health systems between the often short-term goals of donors – who require quick and measurable results on their investments – and the longer-term concerns of health system stewards. That tension has only heightened in recent years, where the surge in international aid for particular diseases has come with ambitious coverage targets and intense scale-up efforts oriented much more to short- than long-term goals (85;86). Though additional funding is particularly welcome in low-income contexts, it can often greatly reduce the negotiating power of national health system stewards in modifying proposed interventions or requesting simultaneous independent evaluations of these interventions as they roll out. In many countries,

Though additional funding is particularly welcome in low-income contexts, it can often greatly reduce the negotiating power of national health system stewards in modifying proposed interventions or requesting simultaneous independent evaluations of these interventions as they roll out.

harmonizing the policies, priorities and perspectives of donors with those of national policy-makers is an immediate and pressing concern – though with few apparent solutions.

For example, there is increasing evidence that while funds for AIDS, TB and Malaria are indeed saving lives (87), they typically come without sufficient strengthening of health systems to sustain these gains. In addition it is increasingly argued that the selective nature of these funding mechanisms (e.g. targeting only specific diseases and subsequent support strategies) may undermine progress towards the long-term goals of effective, high-quality and inclusive health systems (86;88;89). Even where this funding has strengthened components of the health system specifically linked to service delivery in disease prevention and control – such as specific on-the-job staff training – recent research suggests that the selective nature of these health systems strengthening strategies has sometimes been unsustainable, interruptive, and duplicative, putting great strains on the already limited and over-stretched health workforce (84;86;88;90;91). Additionally, focusing on "rapid-impact" treatment interventions for specific diseases and ignoring investments in prevention may also send sharply negative effects across the system's building blocks, including, paradoxically, deteriorating outcomes on the targeted diseases themselves (88).

Many of these issues have been recognized internationally, and a number of donors have agreed to better harmonize their efforts and align with country-led priorities – as outlined in 2005's Paris Declaration on Aid Effectiveness (92). However, a 2008 report showed that, although some progress has been made in applying the Paris Declaration principles, it has been slow and uneven (85). For example, the report found little evidence that donors had improved or made use of existing structures or health information system of recipient countries – and in some cases had even created parallel systems to collect the data they needed. This often creates inefficiency and duplications, and fails to harmonize and use data locally or empower countries to strengthen their own Health Information Systems. Similar negative effects have also been suggested in other parts of the health system, for instance in the areas of finance, service delivery and medical technologies (89).

Change in the process and the nature of the relationship between donors and countries requires time, focused attention at all levels, and a determined political will. *"This means more than just putting more pressure on the gas pedal. It requires a shifting of gears"*(85). And there are indeed some early signs that the gears are shifting. For instance, several funding bodies – e.g. the Global Alliance for Vaccines and Immunization (GAVI) and the Global Fund to Fight AIDS, Tuberculosis and Malaria (GFATM) – have agreed to give health system strengthening greater prominence within their disease-specific initiatives. This should allow for greater flexibility in using their funds to strengthen health systems, even if they still require that activities are tightly linked to their specific health outcomes of interest (84;86). However, recipient countries have so far been slow to request these funds for systems strengthening. Out of US$4.2 billion of Global Fund resources earmarked for health systems strengthening since 2007 – such as building infrastructure, improving laboratories and the development and support of monitoring and evaluation systems – only US$660 million has actually been committed for "cross-cutting" health system strengthening actions that apply to more than one of the three diseases (93). This may perhaps reflect similar issues at the country level – those applying for funds for disease-specific programmes may not work closely with those seeking to strengthen health systems as a whole.

It is here where the systems perspective can best support health systems stewards. If donors are increasingly committed to health system strengthening, then system stewards must maximize this opportunity. The "Ten Steps to Systems Thinking" can usefully guide and frame discussions between system stewards and donors, and lay the groundwork for a system strengthening initiative that all can agree on. Steps 1 (convene stakeholders) and 2 (collectively brainstorm) in particular can address existing paradigms and the new relationships required to transcend them. System stewards must lead discussions among concerned stakeholders – domestic and international – on the merits of different interventions, but also in assessing the potential effects of the intervention on each health systems building block and ensuring that evaluations of these interventions are undertaken as soon as they are rolled out. Strong national governance through the leadership of health systems stewards is central in overcoming the existing set of relationships between funders and recipients.

2. Managing and coordinating partnerships and expectations among system stakeholders

"Donor collaboration has aimed at harmonizing data tools for use at facilities and designing new forms for use in the health management information systems. Even so, reports suggest that the donors have been competing with each other to get results attributed to their own funds, creating a burden on health workers" (91).

While building and supporting partnerships is at the heart of applying a systems perspective to strengthening health systems, managing and coordinating those partnerships – and their expectations – when designing interventions and appraising evaluation findings can pose a daunting challenge. Different partners will have different mandates, priorities and perspectives, all of which may be legitimate. The particular challenge facing health systems stewards lies in effectively managing stakeholder participation and contributions to the design and evaluation of these interventions, ensuring their expectations are met and the process is "owned" without compromising objectivity or the needs of the system itself.

For instance, donors are often caught between their need to demonstrate rapid progress and success in the implementation of funded interventions and their commitment to strengthening the health systems of recipient countries (85). Several recent reports have shown positive signs of increased donor collaboration in the area of health information systems, particularly in harmonizing data tools for use at the facility level – for instance in monitoring patients on antiretroviral treatment (ART) (24;91). However, some countries have experienced difficulties in managing competition among donors and governments in attributing actual outcomes (e.g. number of people on ART)

to their own funding. *"This created a huge problem,"* stated a staff member of Uganda's Ministry of Health, with *"too much double counting"* (91).

Developing and maintaining a culture of open and effective partnerships among a variety of national and international stakeholders is sensible practice for health system stewards. They can provide this leadership by emphasizing the systems perspective for interventions in the health system; by fostering open discussions and transparency in expressing competing objectives and mandates; and by providing the right incentives for data sharing and reconciliation.

3. Implementing and fostering ownership of interventions at the national and sub-national level

"Implementers of policies influence how policies are experienced and their impacts achieved. … the apparently powerless implementers, at the interface between bureaucracy and citizenry, are difficult to control because they have a high margin of discretion in their personal interactions with clients, allowing them to reshape policy in unexpected ways" (46).

As discussed in Chapter 2, one of the main challenges facing a complex system is policy resistance, where seemingly obvious solutions may fail or worsen the situation they were designed to address (43). Research in the United Republic of Tanzania explored this phenomenon in understanding why the implementation rates of community health insurance funds saw less than 10% enrollment after 10 years of implementation (46). The authors showed that the actions of district managers influenced how the policy was translated to implementation, directly contributing to the low implementation rates. Interviews with district managers revealed their underlying reluctance to implement and support the new policy. They judged it as difficult to implement, and blamed the central government for not addressing its financial sustainability. Although district managers were well aware of the policy, they often ignored it and did not view it as part of their mandated district activities. Instead, they saw it as an additional and separate activity operating with its own funds – "like an NGO," as one manager remarked. Consequently, district funds were not mobilized to provide the necessary infrastructure for the community health funds, which led to little public awareness of the programme, and no criteria or guidelines for fee exemption.

Further analysis revealed that district managers felt they had little time to prepare for these activities and described the introduction of the CHF as overly rushed. *"The CHF came to us like a fire brigade,"* reported one of the ward-level interviewees. *"The programme is good but implementation is beset with problems."* These observations were consistent with interviews at the national level describing the considerable political pressure to implement the intervention after promises had been made during an election campaign.

There are several other manifestations of this phenomenon (94-96). South Africa's slow progress in reducing maternal mortality despite more than a decade of intensified efforts have partly been attributed to the practices of health care workers (94), who have reacted in unexpected ways to ongoing structural and financial reforms in the public sector. While the government saw these reforms as a means to improve financial management and health care, front-line health workers perceived a very different set of meanings. They saw little value in the reform policies, feeling stress and fear that any mistakes would lead to their own imprisonment. They saw the policies as unilateral power over them, exerted from above, that made their leaders look good, predominantly at their own expense (94).

The coping behaviour of "street-level" policy implementers (See Box 4.3 for a definition) frustrated with top-down decision-making processes also reflects a lack of local ownership of the policy (97). Clearly some stakeholders essential to implementing an intervention had not been involved in its design. Overcoming the resistance of these implementers comes with understanding and incorporating their perspective – early and adequately. In calling for a multi-stakeholder approach to the design and evaluation of system-level interventions, the systems perspective seeks to give voice to those who are absolutely critical to implementation processes. Indeed, multi-stakeholder involvement is a crucial element throughout the "Ten Steps to Systems Thinking": identifying and involving key stakeholders concerned with or affected by the intervention's implementation is essential, particularly throughout Steps 1-4.

BOX 4.3 DEFINING "STREET-LEVEL" POLICY IMPLEMENTERS

"Street-level" policy implementers – or "street-level bureaucrats" as used in the field of sociology (97) – is a term for those "service providers who work at the implementation end of policies that they have not designed, and who use the degree of relative autonomy that they possess to reinterpret these policies and to revise guidelines according to their own priorities"(96).

4. Building capacity at the country level to apply a systems analytic perspective

"Strengthening research capacity in developing countries is one of the most powerful, cost-effective, and sustainable means of advancing health and development" (98)

Health systems strengthening efforts in developing countries often encounter one or more central capacity constraints: limited multi-disciplinary technical skills compounded by weak research partnerships and collaborations; poor quality and availability of data (75;99); the lack of innovative research methods (100); and limited skills in building and managing partnerships. These problems are deepened by the fact that resources for capacity building are still mainly driven by international sources, providing little or no leverage for developing countries on the selection of priorities for research or skill development or on the proportional use of resources for capacity building (100-102). *"Anyway … it is the donors who decide what the money is spent on … so why set priorities?"* is a common sentiment among developing country researchers (103). However, the ability of country teams to undertake research and analyse their own data is crucial for understanding what works, for whom, and under what circumstances – and for monitoring and addressing problems along the way (100).

Limited multi-disciplinary skills and weak research partnerships and collaborations

While there are indeed some strong research skills in developing countries, many researchers tend to operate in disciplinary "silos," with little institutional incentive to undertake collaborative, multi-disciplinary projects and approaches. The absence of these essential in-country

partnerships is mirrored at the international level. Robust, multi-disciplinary international partnerships between research institutions – often hugely successful – require a substantial investment of time and resources, and as such are typically not encouraged by funders or embedded within institutional reward systems in the developed world (104). Though there are some notable examples of thriving 'North-South' collaborations and capacity building initiatives (100;103;105;106), many research funding bodies still do not see these collaborations as a priority (100;105). Without this funding for collaboration, and without increased investments from domestic sources, existing capacity constraints will continue as a significant drag on health systems strengthening, including diminished leadership roles in intervention design and evaluation, and weak ownership and relevance of the generated information for policy-making (100;102). An encouraging sign for increased domestic efforts to strengthen local capacity to generate and use evidence from research is the recent announcement by the President of the United Republic of Tanzania to triple domestic resources currently spent on science and technology (from 0.3% to 1% of GNP) (103).

Poor data availability and quality

Evaluations of complex health systems interventions depend on a wide range of functional data platforms and monitoring systems to provide up-to-date information on all sub-systems, as well as relevant contextual factors (such as other ongoing health or health-related initiatives). Basic routine data collection systems, including the health information system, procurement and supply chain management data, and financial management systems are still weak and disconnected in many countries, often storing limited and incomplete information (91). Good quality in-country databases for even basic health service reporting are also often lacking (24). This is a crucial barrier, not only for high quality evaluations, but also for monitoring and evaluating the health system's basic functions. Investing in data availability, quality and use is a long-term prospect, but critical to more efficient and coordinated efforts in improving health and health systems. It would also reduce the burden on the already over-stretched health workforce by avoiding short-term "solutions" that create parallel systems (91).

Need for innovative methods

Another more global challenge is the need for new methods development better suited to the complex nature of health systems interventions (100). For example, while capacity for conducting household surveys may exist in some countries (e.g. through Demographic and Health Surveys and other ongoing community-based surveillance systems), capacity for conducting qualitative research is typically less developed. Even in cases where sufficient qualitative skills exist in-country, the focus has traditionally been in using these skills in small-scale studies involving local communities, and much less for complex health systems issues (107;108). Encouraging the development and publication of studies using innovative methods applicable to complex interventions with system-wide effects is critical to increasing the evidence and improving the quality of this body of knowledge. This calls for increased support for this type of research, both in terms of funding and setting research priorities.

Learning skills in building and managing partnerships

Building and managing partnerships is essential to the systems perspective, as illustrated above. This involves specialized skills such as the facilitation of interdisciplinary meetings and discussions involving complex group dynamics, different perspectives and motivations; consensus building without excluding different views; and most importantly, instilling ownership of the eventual products and processes. These skills and techniques are not typically taught in formal institutions and usually require hired external support to lead or impart them. Comprehensive and accessible information on the available resources to acquire these skills, and whether there is a need for additional resources to meet the partnership-building needs of systems stewards, is a top priority.

Part II: Innovative approaches to applying the systems perspective

While the challenges to applying a systems perspective are indeed pressing, and a full understanding of its utility still in its infancy, there are nonetheless some vital opportunities for advancing this approach, and examples demonstrating its value. Key developments over the past several years have explored and highlighted the many possibilities of a systems perspective. These include:

- convening multiple constituencies to conceptualize, design and evaluate different strategies;

- applying the whole systems view;

- developing knowledge translation processes; and

- encouraging an increased national understanding of health systems research and increased global support for strengthening capacity in health systems research.

1. Convening multiple constituencies to conceptualize, design and evaluate different strategies

Chapter 3 argued for the importance of consulting and involving a wide range of stakeholders in the design of system-level interventions and interventions with system-wide effects. This process can elicit valuable insights on the possible synergies and negative ramifications of the proposed intervention, and discuss ways of amplifying or mitigating these effects – either at the design stage or during its implementation and evaluation. Most importantly, however, this multi-stakeholder process fosters strong partnerships and a community of stakeholders addressing an issue collectively, a cohesion and solidarity that itself has strong system-wide effects.

Of course, involving a large number of stakeholders with different views and mandates is far from simple. The convening and brainstorming process is often time-consuming, politically sensitive and may not in the end lead to effective or genuine partnerships unless there are compelling and common goals.

BOX 4.4   INITIATIVE ON THE STUDY AND IMPLEMENTATION OF SYSTEMS (ISIS)

The National Cancer Institute in the United States of America funded this project to examine how systems thinking in tobacco control and public health might be applied. Using many different systems-oriented approaches and methodologies, ISIS was a transdisciplinary effort linking tobacco-control stakeholders and systems experts. ISIS undertook a range of exploratory projects and case studies to assess the potential for systems thinking in tobacco control. ISIS concluded its work with a set of expert consensus guidelines for the future implementation of systems thinking and systems perspectives.

Source: Greater than the Sum: Systems thinking in tobacco control, 2007 (22).

One successful example of multiple constituencies successfully conceptualizing, designing and evaluating different strategies is that of the Initiative on the Study and Implementation of Systems (ISIS) (see Box 4.4). These projects created a multi-stakeholder core to enhance an understanding of the factors affecting tobacco use and to inform decision-making on the most effective strategies to address these factors (29). Aware of the promise – and necessity – of a systems perspective in unraveling and mapping the truly complex and diverse factors influencing health and disease, ISIS is one of a handful of initiatives to prioritize the innovative involvement and insights of multiple stakeholders (22).

In recognizing the utility of multi-disciplinary teams in solving complex problems, ISIS employed "concept mapping" – a structured, participatory methodology promoting consultation among diverse stakeholders (109). The process structures brainstorming across a broad spectrum of issues, either in a face-to-face, real-time group process or virtually over the Internet. The next step is to prioritize the issues through individual sorting and rating, and then synthesizing the inputs, presenting the results back to participants using graphically presented conceptual maps.

One of the central promises of the concept mapping approach is its transparency. When widespread Internet access is available to key stakeholders, a larger number of stakeholders can be involved and the results of the ranking exercises can be easily accessed, reviewed – and challenged. This promotes a deeper, richer discussion and likely more buy-in to the process and the way forward.

2. Applying the whole systems view

Another successful example of a systems perspective comes from the UK government's Foresight programme, which explored the issue of obesity and diabetes, and the "whole systems" view around both (34). Noting the ineffectiveness of interventions designed to curb individual obesity and the development of diabetes as a result, the Foresight programme used a systems mapping approach to understand both the biological and the social complexity of obesity, using advice and insights from a large group of experts drawn from multiple disciplines. In a qualitative mapping exercise, these experts ranked the likely impact of different policy options for different scenarios.

The results of the exercise suggested a number of policy responses that, together, could create a positive impact in tackling obesity. However, no single response generated a high impact on obesity prevalence in all scenarios. A diabetes systems map was developed in response, representing a comprehensive "whole systems" view of the determinants of obesity (see the Foresight Programme's report (34) for an illustration of how the developers took into account feedback loops and the interconnectedness between different factors). The process confirmed that obesity is determined by a complex multi-faceted system of determinants, where no single influence dominates. The complexity of the problem requires a mix of responses, and the study concludes that focusing heavily or exclusively on one element of the system is unlikely to bring about the scale of change required.

3. Developing knowledge translation processes

"A little knowledge that acts is worth infinitely more than much knowledge that is idle."
Kahlil Gibran (1883 – 1931)
Poet Philosopher & Artist

Both concept mapping and the whole systems view are cutting-edge approaches to identifying and resolving key system-level issues and challenges. A third comes from the emerging field of knowledge translation (KT) and its investigations into the interface between the research and policy processes. Related to systems thinking, KT is a strong modality in identifying problems, restructuring relationships, and encouraging the active and innovative flow of knowledge – in both developed and developing country contexts.

As with systems thinking, at the heart of KT lie relationships. KT focuses on developing contextualized knowledge bases, convening deliberative dialogues, and strengthening capacity in order to create new and common ground for better relationships and partnerships between researchers and research-users.[3] Such relationships can work to localize and contextualize scientific evidence to respond to local circumstances (110;111); improve the way the system itself produces, manages and uses evidence for decision-making; and, through the mutual identification and production of policy-guided knowledge, create a deeper appreciation of research processes at the policy level (112).

Though this research and policy interface still requires much more study in the developing world (113), a 2002 meta-analysis found "personal contact" to be the main facilitator of these research and policy processes, and its lack as the main barrier (114). Such contact facilitates shared understandings, common approaches to solutions, develops trust and respect, and also lays the groundwork for appreciating and weighting both evidence and policy priorities in an open and transparent fashion (115) – a finding further confirmed in a recent survey of organizations that support the use of research evidence in LMIC policy development (110).

BOX 4.5 MAKING SOUND CHOICES ON EVIDENCE-INFORMED POLICY-MAKING

"Over recent years there has been a proliferation of literature focusing on knowledge and how to get it into health policy and practice (116;117). For example, in the 1990s the 'evidence-based medicine' movement advocated the greater and more direct use of research evidence in the making of clinical decisions, and this was later broadened into a call for more evidence-based policy as opposed to policies determined through conviction or politics. Part of this interest arose from a perception that even when research provides solutions, these are not necessarily translated into policy and practice".

Source: Alliance HPSR Flagship Report, 2007 (118).

In like fashion, the importance of early and close engagement of researchers and policymakers in developing and evaluating new interventions and policies runs throughout systems thinking, featuring in almost every step of the "Ten Steps to Systems

---

[3] For more information, see the Research Matters Knowledge Translation Toolkit, available at: http://www.idrc.ca/research-matters/ev-128908-201-1-DO_TOPIC.html

Thinking" discussed in Chapter 3. With knowledge translation approaches and modalities now proliferating across the globe – including the creation of national-level knowledge translation platforms and institutes[4] – there is great scope for learning, alignment and even hybridization with systems thinking. Where KT works towards both evidence-informed policy-making and policy-informed research, systems thinking advocates for more *system-informed* decisions and processes across the health system. These are highly complex though complementary processes that most certainly require deeper understanding, further analysis and study.

BOX 4.6   INTERACTION BETWEEN RESEARCHERS AND POLICY-MAKERS ON A ROAD TRAFFIC POLICY IN MALAYSIA

In response to the alarming levels of road traffic injuries in Malaysia, the Department of Road Safety within Malaysia's Ministry of Transport decided to develop and implement various programmes and campaigns to address this problem. Even though there was little local evidence to guide actual policy decisions, policy officials had a skeptical view of research, believing it took too much time to conduct. They were also concerned that research might demonstrate little actual impact of their proposed interventions (119). Eventually, however, a team of researchers negotiated a mutually beneficial research programme with the Department of Road Safety – one that satisfied the policy-makers' need to demonstrate action, and one that also produced the necessary evidence for decision-making. Policy-makers saw the field trials of interventions as practical and necessary to addressing the "how-to" questions surrounding implementation. The research-policy partnership determined common goals and objectives, along with specific intervention options.

After some discussion, policy-makers wanted to develop and launch a national campaign to promote the use of "visibility enhancement materials" – reflectors – though the researchers were able to convince policy-makers to first launch a field trial to determine the efficacy of reflectors. Discussion around the benefits of potentially negative research findings with policy-makers was critical in convincing them to invest in research – if it were found that reflectors were not effective, the field test would be much more cost-effective than a failed nation-wide programme. This process has only strengthened the relationship between researchers and policy-makers and provided the basis for future collaborative research into practice in the country (119).

---

[4]   Examples include the Regional East African Community Health Policy Initiative (REACH-Policy) based in Kampala, Uganda; the Zambia Forum for Health Research (ZAMFOHR), based in Lusaka, Zambia; and the Evidence-Informed Policy Network (EVIPNet), a WHO initiative based in Geneva, Switzerland that supports KT in a variety of developing-world contexts.

4. Encouraging an increased national understanding of health systems research and increased global support for strengthening capacity in health systems research

Crucially, systems thinking depends upon an understanding of "the system" among key stakeholders, and a wider appreciation of health systems research. There have been some recent compelling developments in both, particularly in renewed capacity strengthening efforts targeting researchers looking to sharpen their skills in health systems research. These include:

■ the Consortium for Advanced Research Training in Africa (CARTA). Based at the African Population and Health Research Centre in Nairobi, Kenya, CARTA seeks to boost the skills of doctoral students in health research, particularly through the acquisition of multi-disciplinary and KT skills;

■ the Health Research Capacity Strengthening Initiative (HRCS). Now operating in both Kenya and Malawi, HRCS aims to coordinate in-country health research and spearhead capacity-building activities, particularly in promoting career pathways for young researchers.

■ The Initiative to Strengthen Health Research Capacity in Africa (ISHReCA). This network of health researchers looks to radical solutions to strengthen African capacity to conduct health research through new platforms to build and integrate capacity at the individual, institutional and system levels.

Conclusion

There are some formidable challenges facing – and even preventing – the full application of a systems perspective in understanding and solving weaknesses in developing country health systems. This Chapter has discussed some of the more daunting challenges but also highlighted important and innovative systems thinking solutions and achievements. Clearly, there is a great deal of work yet to do, but if systems thinking can turn the spotlight to the leadership and commitment of system stewards, and to new partnerships across the health system – from policy implementers to global funders – then it may very well open the next chapter in strengthening health systems.

Systems thinking, it should be remembered, is not a panacea. It will not solve all of the stark challenges to strengthening health systems in developing countries. However, it is one of several essential tools to restructuring the relationships within the health system. The more often and more comprehensively the actors and parts of the system can talk to each other – communicating, sharing, problem-solving – the better chance any initiative to strengthen health systems has. Real progress will undoubtedly require time (92), significant change, and support for the present momentum to build capacity across the system and to promote multi-stakeholder approaches in the design and evaluation of system-level interventions. However, the change is necessary – and needed now.

5

Systems thinking for health systems strengthening: Moving forward

*"A system just can't respond to short-term changes
when it has long-term delays. That's why a massive
central-planning system ... necessarily functions poorly"*.
Donella Meadows, 1999 (53).

The growing focus
on health systems

It has become commonplace in health development and global health initiatives to experience "system-wide barriers" to rapid attainment of global goals for health. Indeed, the weak performance of many health systems to deliver disease- or programme-specific goals continues to reinforce vertical solutions that bypass systems. Yet the stewards of national health systems must deal daily with their real-world challenges to build effective, efficient, equitable and sustainable systems to ensure national health goals. Fortunately everyone agrees that both trajectories (vertical and horizontal) are focused on the same end, and that bringing them into a single coherent approach would be mutually beneficial. Most global health initiatives now recognize the need to invest in health system strengthening as a requisite for success. Most national health system stewards want to leverage such investments in support of system-wide improvements. The question though is how to do this.

In this Report, we promote systems thinking as a core approach to understand how health interventions exert their system-wide effects and how this systems analysis can be used to better design and evaluate interventions in health systems.

There has never been a better time for applying systems thinking in health systems. Efforts to define health systems (83) have resulted in comprehensive frameworks for the key elements and building blocks of contemporary health systems (83). Funding for health interventions and for health systems strengthening has increased substantially. Scaling up what works has become a main mandate of health system reforms in developing countries. At the same time, developed country health systems have increasingly adopted systems thinking at sub-system levels to tackle complex and large-scale challenges such as major organizational systems (e.g. hospital systems (121), health information systems (122)) or complex health challenges (e.g. the tobacco (22), diabetes (27) and obesity epidemics (34)). This Report goes further and explores the opportunity to apply systems thinking to the health system as a whole, and particularly to health system strengthening interventions and their evaluation in developing countries.

"The global health agenda is shifting from an emphasis on disease-specific approaches to a focus on strengthening of health systems. ...Yet clearly the disease-focused programmes are concerned about shifts in global resources to health systems." Takemi and Reich, 2009 (120).

In order to introduce systems thinking in a context that is often dominated by single disease and fragmented programme thinking, we have proposed ten sequential steps to begin solving complex system-level problems (see Box 5.1). None of these steps should be alien to any practitioner in health systems research or development. But greater benefits emerge from the synergies generated when *all Ten Steps are conducted in sequence*. Applying the Ten Steps opens the needed space to appreciate and address complexity, connections, feedback loops, time delays and non-linear relationships.

Schools of thought and experience

This Report intends to be a primer and initiation into systems thinking and to open windows on inspiring concepts and experiences. Though much of the systems thinking literature cited may be unfamiliar to many, we encourage readers to examine the provided reference list for deeper insights into the systems thinking approach for health.

There is nothing completely original or unfamiliar in the Ten Steps. Some developing country system stewards may well be employing some or even all of the Ten Steps, using multi-disciplinary and multi-stakeholder teams. Rather than proposing something that is totally new, this Report aims to make system-wide approaches with all steps in sequence the norm – rather than the exception – and to promote better documentation of those instances where system-wide approaches to design and evaluation have indeed been used. That said, examples of health system strengthening that deliberately intervene simultaneously in all six building blocks of a health system are uncommon, though when this has happened large synergistic effects have resulted (Box 5.2). Evaluating such effects in relation to a suite of interventions demands a full systems thinking approach, not just to the interventions, but also to the evaluation itself.

BOX 5.2 EXAMPLE OF SYSTEM-WIDE EFFECTS OF A SYSTEM-WIDE INTERVENTION

Health system strengthening interventions rarely include a suite of interventions applied simultaneously to target each building block of the health system. One example of this is the Tanzania Ministry of Health Essential Health Interventions Project (TEHIP). Launched in 1996, TEHIP led to large synergistic health effects at the district level (123). It targeted the **Governance** building block through district decentralization and increased ownership of the planning process and fiscal resources; **Financing** through providing an untied district-level SWAp (Sector Wide Approach) basket fund and through a district health accounts tool for resource allocation; **Information** through providing annual district health profiles founded on community-based sentinel surveillance systems and through radios to improve communications among health facilities and managers; **Human Resources** through empowering use of local basket funds for management training, communications, and other means to improve team work and working conditions for new health interventions; **Medicines and Technologies** through the ability to solve drug stock-outs by accessing the local basket fund and increased authority to spend; and **Service Delivery** through early adoption of new interventions such as Integrated Management of Childhood Illness and Insecticide Treated Bed Nets.

All interventions were highly interdependent. The financing intervention was essential – but funding alone would not have lead to such good performance outcomes (including a 40% drop in under-five mortality seen within five years). Without the governance change allowing decentralization of responsibility with greater authority for spending, little would have changed. Without the new information sources that related spending priorities to health priorities, the subsequent resource re-allocations (which resulted in service delivery change) would not have occurred. Without the feedback on progress from their information system, there would have been little idea of what was working, and what not. Without further governance changes allowing ownership of planning and the flexibility to spend on human resource training, the new and more powerful interventions would not have been adopted so quickly.

It is impossible to say which of the interventions in this web were the most important. The evaluation used a multi-institutional, multi-disciplinary, plausibility design that provided compelling information for districts and policy-makers. Tanzania's Ministry of Health scaled up many of the innovations and lessons learnt in TEHIP in 2000 with similar strong effects seen at the national level by 2004 (124).

In this Report, we have taken the case of a major contemporary system-level intervention to show how – using the first four of the Ten Steps – a stronger partnership of stakeholders can deliver a richer understanding of the implications of the intervention. This in turn creates a greater sense of ownership, and a more robust intervention design with a greater chance to maximize synergies and mitigate unintended negative effects. The remaining steps illustrate how the research and evaluation community can contribute to verify the design and fine-tune it over time. Such approaches to intervention and evaluation are infrequent, and when proposed, are rarely funded. So what is the way forward in mainstreaming the systems perspective?

Moving forward

Not surprisingly, practitioners of systems thinking have considered the actions required to build capacity for the systems perspective. These typically centre on the creation of a systems thinking environment conducive to a strong orientation to team science and development. The approaches generally include: developing and applying systems methods and processes; building system knowledge capacity; building and maintaining network relationships; and encouraging a systems culture (29).

There are, of course, practical challenges to introducing and applying systems thinking in the health sector (33). Systems thinkers have conceptually mapped these. They include the need to work along the following lines:

1) explore problems from a systems perspective;

2) show potentials of solutions that work across sub-systems;

3) promote dynamic networks of diverse stakeholders;

4) inspire learning; and

5) foster more system-wide planning, evaluation and research.

For the community that this Report primarily addresses (health system stewards, researchers and funders interested in health systems strengthening in low-income settings) the following are some reflections on possible actions or next steps to deepen and develop systems thinking for health systems strengthening.

Task Force on Systems Thinking for Health Systems. Extending a systems thinking movement and culture requires a number of combined initiatives. Convening a temporary task force or think tank engaging key practitioners from the health systems thinking community – together with key stakeholders for health system strengthening – may be one way to achieve this. Such a Task Force could, for example, be convened under the auspices of the WHO Health Systems Department and the Alliance for Health Policy and Systems Research with the support of other interested parties.

Systems Thinking network or communities of practice. A natural spin-off from the Task Force would be the development of a network or community of practice around systems thinking for health systems. These would of course include country implementers and donors. This could deepen the skills of systems thinking, enable strong horizontal learning among systems thinkers, be a resource for newcomers, and fine-tune the Ten Steps. Emerging networks could tackle many of the issues listed below.

Building the capacity of system stewards. A special case of the community of practice might be the issue of building capacity among policy-makers for systems thinking. This could entail the creation of policy briefs or briefing notes that provide short, digestible descriptions of best practice. One of the core actions of the Task Force, and supported by members of the networks, could be developing capacity-building courses for system stewards which could draw upon other successful models of training policy-makers (e.g. the Executive Training for Research Application (EXTRA) programme offered by the Canadian Health Services Research Foundation).

Systems Thinking conference for best practices. There is a growing body of experience in applying systems thinking at the sub-system or building-block level, but no international forum to bring those experiences together in a peer environment for further development and catalysis. A conference or similar event could be an early action supported by the Task Force or networks, to further convene the community of practice to focus in particular on sharing experiences and methods development.

Systems Thinking methods. Continued development of conceptual approaches and methods is a constant need. The Task Force, networks and conference will be critical to identifying these needs, breaking down the "silos," and driving the development agenda forward.

Health systems dynamic modeling. There is increasing interest and activity in dynamic modeling to forecast the effects of new health interventions in disease-specific contexts (e.g. malaria vaccines) (125;126). The larger these modeling projects become, the more the modelers realize they must integrate modeling of health service delivery and health systems. This greatly increases the complexity of their models, but will be of particular use to the systems dynamics and modeling demands of system thinking. These efforts could be networked and could contribute immensely to health system design (33;127).

Expanding Systems Thinking in schools of public health and degrees in health systems management. Some schools of international public health have already started to introduce systems theory in their curricula. The communities of practice as presented above may support and promote these programs for a new generation of public health expertise.

Applying the Ten Steps. A consortium of health system stakeholders, researchers and development donors could be assembled for testing the Ten Steps proposed here with regard to the large new initiatives that are emerging for health systems strengthening initiatives (e.g. from the G8, International Health Partnership+, Global Fund to fight AIDS, Tuberculosis and Malaria, Global Alliance for Vaccines and Immunization, and so on).

A Journal of Systems Thinking for Health. There are very few open-source, peer-reviewed journals dedicated to health systems development. Moreover, health systems research of the nature demanded by systems thinking (for example when multiple interventions with multiple effects are to be described) will suffer from the publication bias against long papers. This also affects health systems research from a systems-wide perspective. A dedicated journal for health systems with a focus on Systems Thinking for Health will be a timely addition.

Wrapping up

These are exciting times for health systems strengthening. The opportunities are immense, yet so too are the challenges. More of the same will not suffice to achieve the ambitious goals that have been set. Beyond system-centered approaches, we need continual innovation – achieved not through a radical departure from the past but by creatively combining past experience. This Report contributes to this effort by exploring the huge potential of systems thinking in designing our way forward to stronger health systems, and to evaluating how that progress is achieved. The Report identifies systems thinking as a hugely valuable but under-exploited approach. We introduce the concepts, and discuss what they can mean for health systems strengthening. We draw on emerging successes from the application of systems thinking at smaller scales and propose ways in which it can be applied at the scales now being addressed in many developing country health systems. We have shown what it might look like using illustrations from highly contemporary interventions. We have explored the challenges and sketch some steps for the way forward to harness these approaches and link them to these emerging opportunities.

Future health systems will undoubtedly be anchored in dynamic, strongly designed, and decidedly systemic architecture. These will be systems capable of high performance in producing health with equity. The question is how to accelerate progress to that end. We hope this Report of the Alliance stimulates both fresh thinking and concrete action towards such stronger health systems.

As always, the final message is to the funders of health system strengthening and health systems research who will need to recognize the potential in these opportunities, be prepared to take risks in investing in such innovations, and play an active role in both driving and following this agenda towards more systemic and evidence-informed health development.

Reference List

(1) United Nations. *The Millennium Development Goals Report 2009.* New York, United Nations, 2009.

(2) Bryce J et al. Countdown to 2015: tracking intervention coverage for child survival. *Lancet*, 2006, 368(9541):1067-1076.

(3) Victora CG et al. Co-coverage of preventive interventions and implications for child-survival strategies: evidence from national surveys. *Lancet*, 2005, 366(9495):1460-1466.

(4) Kruk ME, Freedman LP. Assessing health system performance in developing countries: A review of the literature. *Health Policy*, 2007, 85(3): 263-276.

(5) World Health Organization. *Everybody's Business: Strengthening Health Systems to Improve Health Outcomes: WHO's Framework for Action.* Geneva, WHO, 2007.

(6) Travis P et al. Overcoming health-systems constraints to achieve the Millennium Development Goals. *Lancet*, 2004, 364(9437):900-906.

(7) Tugwell P et al. Applying clinical epidemiological methods to health equity: the equity effectiveness loop. *BMJ*, 2006, 332(7537):358-361.

(8) World Health Organization Maximizing Positive Synergies Collaborative Group. An assessment of interactions between global health initiatives and country health systems. *Lancet*, 2009, 373(9681):2137-2169.

(9) Banati P, Moatti JP. The positive contributions of global health initiatives. *Bulletin of the World Health Organization*, 2008, 86(11):820.

(10) Yu D et al. Investment in HIV/AIDS programs: Does it help strengthen health systems in developing countries? *Globalization and Health*, 2008, 4:8.

(11) Hanefeld J. How have Global Health Initiatives impacted on health equity? *Promotion & Education*, 2008, 15(1):19-23.

(12) Schieber GJ et al. Financing global health: mission unaccomplished. *Health Affairs*, 2007, 26(4):921-934.

(13) Murray CJ, Frenk J, Evans T. The Global Campaign for the Health MDGs: challenges, opportunities, and the imperative of shared learning. *Lancet*, 2007, 370(9592):1018-1020.

(14) Buse K, Walt G. Globalisation and multi-lateral public-private health partnerships: issues for health policy. In: K Lee, S Fustukian, K Buse, editors. *Health Policy in a Globalising World.* Cambridge, Cambridge University Press, 2007.

(15) Lu C et al. Absorptive capacity and disbursements by the Global Fund to Fight AIDS, Tuberculosis and Malaria: analysis of grant implementation. *Lancet*, 2006, 368(9534):483-488.

(16) Labonte R, Schrecker T. The G8 and global health: What now? What next? *Canadian Journal of Public Health*, 2006, 97(1):35-38.

(17) Pawson R et al. Realist review – a new method of systematic review designed for complex policy interventions. *Journal of Health Services Research & Policy*, 2005, 10 Suppl 1:21-34.

(18) Golden BR, Martin RL. Aligning the stars: Using systems thinking to (re)design Canadian healthcare. *Healthcare Quarterly*, 2004, 7(4):34-42.

(19) Plsek PE, Greenhalgh T. Complexity science: The challenge of complexity in health care. *BMJ*, 2001, 323(7313):625-628.

(20) World Health Organization. *People at the centre of health care: harmonizing mind and body, people and systems.* Geneva, WHO, 2007.

(21) World Health Organization. *Primary Health Care: Now more than ever.* Geneva, WHO, 2008.

(22) Best A et al. *Greater than the sum: Systems thinking in tobacco control.* Bethesda, MD, National Cancer Institute, US Department of Health and Human Services, National Institutes of Health, 2007.

(23) Office of Social and Behavioural Sciences Research. *Contributions of Behavioral and Social Sciences Research to Improving the Health of the Nation: A Prospectus for the Future.* US Department of Health and Human Services, National Institutes of Health, 2007.

(24) Health Metrics Network. *Framework and standards for country health information systems.* 2nd ed. Geneva, World Health Organization, 2008.

(25) Craig P et al. Developing and evaluating complex interventions: the new Medical Research Council guidance. *BMJ* 2008, 337:a1655.

(26) Shiell A, Hawe P, Gold L. Complex interventions or complex systems? Implications for health economic evaluation. *BMJ*, 2008, 336(7656):1281-1283.

(27) Kalim K, Carson E, Cramp D. An illustration of whole systems thinking. *Health Services Management Research*, 2006, 19(3):174-185.

(28) Richmond B. The "thinking" in systems thinking: *Seven essential skills*. Waltham MA, Pegasus Communications, 2000.

(29) Leischow SJ et al. Systems thinking to improve the public's health. *American Journal of Preventive Medicine*, 2008, 35(2 Suppl):S196-S203.

(30) Pickett RB, Kennedy MM. Systems thinking and managing complexity, Part two. *Clinical Leadership Management Review*, 2003, 17(2):103-107.

(31) Pickett RB, Kennedy MM. Systems thinking and managing complexity, Part One. *Clinical Leadership Management Review*, 2003, 17(1):34-38.

(32) Sterman JD. Learning from evidence in a complex world. *American Journal of Public Health*, 2006, 96(3):505-514.

(33) Trochim WM et al. Practical challenges of systems thinking and modeling in public health. *American Journal of Public Health*, 2006, 96(3):538-546.

(34) Butland B et al. *Foresight: Tackling Obesities: Future Choices*. London, UK Government Office for Science, 2007.

(35) Finegood DT, Karanfil O, Matteson CL. Getting from analysis to action: Framing obesity research, policy and practice with a solution-oriented complex systems lens. *Healthcare Papers*, 2008, 9(1):36-41.

(36) Shiell A. The danger in conservative framing of a complex, systems-level issue. *Healthcare Papers*, 2008, 9(1):42-45.

(37) Atun R, Menabde N. Health systems and systems thinking. In: Coker R, Atun R, McKee M, editors. *Health systems and the challenge of communicable disease: Experience from Europe and Latin America.* Berkshire, Open University Press, 2009: 122-140.

(38) Holden LM. Complex adaptive systems: concept analysis. *Journal of Advanced Nursing*, 2005, 52(6):651-657.

(39) Rickles D, Hawe P, Shiell A. A simple guide to chaos and complexity. *Journal of Epidemiology and Community Health*, 2007, 61(11):933-937.

(40) Bierema LL. Systems thinking: a new lens for old problems. *Journal of Continuing Education in the Health Professions,* 2003, 23 Suppl 1:S27-S33.

(41) World Bank. *Healthy Development: The World Bank Strategy for Health Nutrition and Population Results: Annex L.* World Bank, 2007.

(42) Meadows D, Richardson J, Bruckmann G. *Groping in the dark: the first decade of global modelling.* New York, NY, Wiley, 1982.

(43) Meadows D. *Thinking in systems: A primer.* White River, VT, Sustainability Institute, 2008.

(44) The Lancet. Data fraud in: This week in Medicine. *Lancet*, 2009, 373[9671], 1222.

(45) Adam T et al. Capacity constraints to the adoption of new interventions: consultation time and the integrated management of childhood illness in Brazil. *Health Policy & Planning*, 2004, 20(Suppl 1):i49-i57.

(46) Kamuzora P, Gilson L. Factors influencing implementation of the Community Health Fund in Tanzania. *Health Policy & Planning*, 2007, 22(2):95-102.

(47) International Health Partnership. *Annual Monitoring and Evaluation of the International Health Partnership & related Initiatives (IHP+).* WHO, 2009.

(48) Shiell A, Riley T. Theorizing interventions as events in systems. *American Journal of Community Psychology*, 2009, 43(3):267-276.

(49) Hawe P, Bond L, Butler L. Knowledge theories can inform evaluation practice. What can a complexity lens add? *New Directions in Evaluation*, 2009; in press.

(50) Hawe P, Ghali L. Use of social network analysis to map the social relationships of staff and teachers at school. *Health Education Research*, 2008, 23(1):62-69.

(51) Hawe P et al. Methods for exploring implementation variation and local context within a cluster randomised community intervention trial. *Journal of Epidemiology and Community Health*, 2004, 58(9):788-793.

(52) O'Conner J, McDermott I. *The Art of Systems Thinking: Essential Skills for Creativity and Problem-Solving.* San Francisco, CA, Thorsons Publishing, 1997.

(53) Meadows D. *Leverage Points: Places to Intervene in a System*. White River, VT, The Sustainability Institute, 1999.

(54) Leischow SJ, Milstein B. Systems thinking and modeling for public health practice. *American Journal of Public Health*, 2006, 96(3):403-405.

(55) Atun RA et al. Introducing a complex health innovation – primary health care reforms in Estonia (multimethods evaluation). *Health Policy*, 2006, 79(1):79-91.

(56) Atun RA et al. Diffusion of complex health innovations – implementation of primary health care reforms in Bosnia and Herzegovina. *Health Policy & Planning*, 2007, 22(1):28-39.

(57) Campbell NC et al. Designing and evaluating complex interventions to improve health care. *BMJ*, 2007, 334(7591):455-459.

(58) Craig P et al. *Developing and evaluating complex interventions: new guidance.* Medical Research Council, 2009.

(59) Casalino LP et al. Will pay-for-performance and quality reporting affect health care disparities? *Health Affairs*, 2007, 26(3):w405-w414.

(60) Eichler R. Can Pay for Performance increase utilisation by the poor and improve quality of health services. Discussion Paper. Washington DC, Centre for Global Development, 2006.

(61) Johannes L et al. *Performance-based contracting in health. The experience in three projects in Africa.* OBA Approaches [19]. The Global Partnership for Output-based Aid, 2009.

(62) Liu X, Mills A. The influence of bonus payments to doctors on hospital revenue: results of a quasi-experimental study. *Applied Health Economics and Health Policy*, 2003, 2(2):91-98.

(63) Soeters R, Habineza C, Peerenboom PB. Performance-based financing and changing the district health system: experience from Rwanda. *Bulletin of the World Health Organization*, 2006, 84(11):884-889.

(64) Lagarde M, Haines A, Palmer N. Conditional cash transfers for improving uptake of health interventions in low- and middle-income countries: a systematic review. *JAMA*, 2007, 298(16):1900-1910.

(65) Brugha R, Varvasovszky Z. Stakeholder analysis: a review. *Health Policy & Planning*, 2000, 15(3):239-246.

(66) Schmeer K. *Stakeholder analysis guidelines*. Bethesda, USA, Abt Associates, 1999.

(67) Campbell M et al. Framework for design and evaluation of complex interventions to improve health. *BMJ*, 2000, 321:694-696.

(68) Graham A et al. Translating cancer control research into primary care practice: a conceptual framework. *American Journal of Lifestyle Medicine*, 2008, 2:241-248.

(69) Victora CG et al. Context matters: interpreting impact findings in child survival evaluations. *Health Policy & Planning*, 2005, 20(suppl_1):i18-i31.

(70) Baltussen R, Leidl R, Ament A. Real world designs in economic evaluation. Bridging the gap between clinical research and policy-making. *Pharmacoeconomics*, 1999, 16(5 Pt 1):449-458.

(71) Lemmer B, Grellier R, Steven J. Systematic review of nonrandom and qualitative research literature: exploring and uncovering an evidence base for health visiting and decision making. *Qualitative Health Research*, 1999, 9(3):315-328.

(72) Hawe P, Shiell A, Riley T. Complex interventions: how "out of control" can a randomised controlled trial be? *BMJ*, 2004, 328(7455):1561-1563.

(73) Bonell CP et al. Alternatives to randomisation in the evaluation of public-health interventions: design challenges and solutions. *Journal of Epidemiology and Community Health*, 2009 [epub ahead of print].

(74) King G et al. Public policy for the poor? A randomised assessment of the Mexican universal health insurance programme. *Lancet*, 2009, 373(9673):1447-1454.

(75) Black N. Why we need observational studies to evaluate the effectiveness of health care. *BMJ*, 1996, 312:1215-1218.

(76) Smith PG, Morrow RH. *Field trials of health interventions in developing countries*. 2nd Edition. London: Macmillan, 1996.

(77) Habicht JP, Victora CG, Vaughan JP. Evaluation designs for adequacy, plausibility and probability of public health programme performance and impact. *International Journal of Epidemiology*, 1999, 28(1):10-18.

(78) Habicht JP, Victora CG, Vaughan JP. *A framework for linking evaluation needs to design choices – with special reference to the fields of health and nutrition*. UNICEF, 1997.

(79) Victora C, Habicht J-P, Bryce J. Evidence-based public health: Moving beyond randomized trials. *American Journal of Public Health*, 2004, 94(3):400-415.

(80) Hanson K et al. Household ownership and use of insecticide treated nets among target groups after implementation of a national voucher programme in the United Republic of Tanzania: plausibility study using three annual cross sectional household surveys. *BMJ*, 2009, 339(jul02_1):b2434.

(81) Hanson K et al. Vouchers for scaling up insecticide-treated nets in Tanzania: Methods for monitoring and evaluation of a national health system intervention. *BMC Public Health*, 2008, 8(1):205.

(82) Richmond B. *Systems Thinking: Four Key Questions*. High Performance Systems Inc., 1991.

(83) World Health Organization. *The World Health Report 2000: Health systems: Improving performance*. Geneva, World Health Organization, 2000.

(84) Hanefeld J, Musheke M. What impact do Global Health Initiatives have on human resources for antiretroviral treatment roll-out? A qualitative policy analysis of implementation processes in Zambia. *Human Resources for Health*, 2009, 7.

(85) Organization for Economic Co-operation and Development. *2008 Survey on Monitoring the Paris Declaration – Making Aid more Effective by 2010*. Paris, OECD, 2009.

(86) Marchal B, Cavalli A, Kegels G. Global Health Actors Claim To Support Health System Strengthening – Is This Reality or Rhetoric? *PLoS Medicine*, 2009, 6(4):1-5.

(87) Samb B et al. An assessment of interactions between global health initiatives and country health systems. *Lancet*, 2009, 373(9681):2137-2169.

(88) Assefa Y et al. Rapid scale-up of antiretroviral treatment in Ethiopia: successes and system-wide effects. *PLoS Medicine*, 2009, 6(4):e1000056.

(89) Biesma RG et al. The effects of global health initiatives on country health systems: a review of the evidence from HIV/AIDS control. *Health Policy & Planning*, 2009, 24(4):239-252.

(90) Travis P, Bennett S, Haines A. Overcoming health-systems constraints to achieve the millennium development goals. *Lancet*, 2005, 365(9456):294.

(91) Oomman N, Bernstein M, Rosenzweig S. *Seizing the opportunity on AIDS and health systems*. Washington DC, Centre for Global Development, 2008.

(92) Organization for Economic Co-operation and Development. *Paris Declaration on Aid Effectiveness*. Paris, OECD, 2005.

(93) Global Fund to fight AIDS, TB and Malaria. *Scaling up for impact: Results report 2008*. Executive summary. Geneva, GFATM, 2009.

(94) Penn-Kekana L, Blaauw D, Schneider H. 'It makes me want to run away to Saudi Arabia': management and implementation challenges for public financing reforms from a maternity ward perspective. *Health Policy & Planning*, 2004, 19:I71-I77.

(95) Walker L, Gilson L. 'We are bitter but we are satisfied': nurses as street-level bureaucrats in South Africa. *Social Science & Medicine*, 2004, 59(6):1251-1261.

(96) Kaler A, Watkins SC. Disobedient distributors: Street-level bureaucrats and would-be patrons in community-based family planning programs in rural Kenya. *Studies in Family Planning*, 2001, 32(3):254-269.

(97) Lipsky M. *Street-level Bureaucracy: Dilemmas of the Individual in Public Services*. New York, Russell Sage Foundation, 1980.

(98) The Commission on Health Research for Development. *Health research: Essential link to equity in development*. New York, Oxford University Press, 1990.

(99) Victora CG, Habicht JP, Bryce J. Evidence-based public health: moving beyond randomized trials. *American Journal of Public Health*, 2004, 94(3):400-405.

(100) Bennett S et al. From Mexico to Mali: progress in health policy and systems research. *Lancet*, 2008, 372(9649):1571-1578.

(101) White F. Capacity-building for health research in developing countries: a manager's approach. *Pan American Journal of Public Health*, 2002, 12(3):165-172.

(102) The Global Ministerial Forum on Research for Health. *The Bamako call to action on research for health*. Geneva, Global Ministerial Forum on Research for Health, 2008.

(103) Council on Health Research for Development (COHRED). *Supporting national health research systems in low and middle income countries. Annual Report 2008*. Geneva, COHRED, 2008.

(104) Harris E. Building scientific capacity in developing countries. *EMBO Reports*, 2004, 5(1):7-11.

(105) Rathgeber EM. *Research partnerships in international health: Capitalizing on opportunity*. Stakeholders' Meeting Berlin, 16-18 March 2009, Research Partnership for Neglected Diseases of Poverty.

(106) International Development Research Centre. *Working together to strengthen skills – IDRC's strategic evaluation of capacity development, phase 3: Developing the framework*. Ottawa, International Development Research Centre, 2007.

(107) Pfeiffer J, Nichter M. What can critical medical anthropology contribute to global health? A health systems perspective. *Medical Anthropology Quarterly*, 2008, 22(4):410-415.

(108) Gilson L, Raphaely N. The terrain of health policy analysis in low and middle income countries: a review of published literature 1994-2007. *Health Policy & Planning*, 2008, 23(5):294-307.

(109) Trochim WMK. An Introduction to Concept Mapping for Planning and Evaluation. *Evaluation and Program Planning*, 1989, 12(1):1-16.

(110) Lavis JN et al. Evidence-informed health policy 4 – Case descriptions of organizations that support the use of research evidence. *Implementation Science*, 2008, 3:56.

(111) Bowen S, Zwi AB. Pathways to "evidence-informed" policy and practice: A framework for action. *PLoS Medicine*, 2005, 2(7):600-605.

(112) Lomas J. Using research to inform healthcare managers' and policy makers' questions: from summative to interpretive synthesis. *Healthcare Policy*, 2005, 1(1):55-71.

(113) Hamid M et al. EVIPNet: translating the spirit of Mexico. *Lancet*, 2005, 366(9499):1758-1760.

(114) Innvaer S et al. Health policy-makers' perceptions of their use of evidence: a systematic review. *Journal of Health Services Research & Policy*, 2002, 7(4):239-244.

(115) Lavis JN et al. Assessing country-level efforts to link research to action. *Bulletin of the World Health Organization*, 2006, 84(8):620-628.

(116) Court J, Hovland I, Young J. *Bridging research and policy in international development*. London, ITDG Publishing, 2004.

(117) Stone D, Maxwell M. *Global Knowledge networks and international development: bridges across boundaries*. Routledge, 2005.

(118) Green A, Sara Bennett, eds. *Sound Choices: enhancing capacity for evidence-informed health policy*. Geneva, Alliance for Health Policy and Systems Research, WHO, 2007.

(119) Hyder AA et al. Integrating ethics, health policy and health systems in low- and middle-income countries: case studies from Malaysia and Pakistan. *Bulletin of the World Health Organization*, 2008, 86(8):606-611.

(120) Reich MR, Takemi K. G8 and strengthening of health systems: follow-up to the Toyako summit. *Lancet*, 2009, 373(9662):508-515.

(121) Holland C, Lien J. Systems thinking: managing the pieces as part of the whole. *Clinical Leadership Management Review*, 2001, 15(3):153-157.

(122) Rothschild AS et al. Leveraging systems thinking to design patient-centered clinical documentation systems. *International Journal of Medical Information*, 2005, 74(5):395-398.

(123) de Savigny D et al. *Fixing Health Systems*. 2nd Edition. Ottawa, International Development Research Centre, 2008.

(124) Masanja H et al. Child survival gains in Tanzania: analysis of data from demographic and health surveys. *Lancet*, 2008, 371(9620):1276-1283.

(125) Homer JB, Hirsch GB. System dynamics modeling for public health: background and opportunities. *American Journal of Public Health*, 2006, 96(3):452-458.

(126) Smith T et al. Towards a comprehensive simulation model of malaria epidemiology and control. *Parasitology*, 2008, 1-10.

(127) Sanderson C, Gruen RL. *Analytical models for decision making*. Open University Press, 2006.

The Alliance gratefully acknowledges funding from the Department for International Development (DFID, United Kingdom), the Australian Government's overseas aid program (AusAID), the International Development Research Center (IDRC, Canada), the Government of Norway, Sida-SAREC (Sweden) and the Wellcome Trust (United Kingdom).

Notes

Notes